A PLUME BOOK

101 WAYS TO SAVE MONEY ON HEALTH CARE

CYNTHIA J. KOELKER, MD, is a board-certified family physician with degrees from MIT, Case Western Reserve University School of Medicine, and the University of Akron. She served in the National Health Service Corps to finance her medical education. She continues to practice medicine in Akron, Ohio.

101 Ways
to Save Money
on Health Care

TIPS TO HELP YOU
SPEND SMART
AND STAY HEALTHY

Cynthia J. Koelker, MD

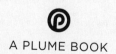

A PLUME BOOK

PLUME
Published by the Penguin Group
Penguin Group (USA) Inc., 375 Hudson Street, New York, New York 10014, U.S.A. ▪ Penguin Group (Canada), 90 Eglinton Avenue East, Suite 700, Toronto, Ontario, Canada M4P 2Y3 (a division of Pearson Penguin Canada Inc.) ▪ Penguin Books Ltd., 80 Strand, London WC2R ORL, England ▪ Penguin Ireland, 25 St. Stephen's Green, Dublin 2, Ireland (a division of Penguin Books Ltd.) ▪ Penguin Group (Australia), 250 Camberwell Road, Camberwell, Victoria 3124, Australia (a division of Pearson Australia Group Pty. Ltd.) ▪ Penguin Books India Pvt. Ltd., 11 Community Centre, Panchsheel Park, New Delhi – 110017, India ▪ Penguin Group (NZ), 67 Apollo Drive, Rosedale, North Shore 0632, New Zealand (a division of Pearson New Zealand Ltd.) ▪ Penguin Books (South Africa) (Pty.) Ltd., 24 Sturdee Avenue, Rosebank, Johannesburg 2196, South Africa.

Penguin Books Ltd., Registered Offices: 80 Strand, London WC2R ORL, England

Published by Plume, a member of Penguin Group (USA) Inc. Previously published by MD Books USA.

First Plume Printing, September 2010

10 9 8 7 6 5 4 3 2 1

℗ REGISTERED TRADEMARK—MARCA REGISTRADA

LIBRARY OF CONGRESS CATALOGING-IN-PUBLICATION DATA

Koelker, Cynthia J.
    101 ways to save money on health care: tips to help you spend smart and stay healthy / Cynthia J. Koelker.
        p. cm.
    Includes index.
    ISBN 978-0-452-29694-7
    1. Medicine, Popular.   2. Medical care, Cost of.   I. Title.   II. Title: One hundred and one ways to save money on health care: tips to help you spend smart and stay healthy.
    RC82.K67 2010
    616—dc22

Printed in the United States of America

PUBLISHER'S NOTE

All brand names, product names, and services used in this book are trademarks, registered trademarks, or trade names of their respective holders. Neither the author nor the publisher is associated with any pharmaceutical company, product, or vendor.

While the author and publisher have been conscientious in preparing this book, it is not meant to offer professional medical advice, and the use of this book does not establish a doctor-patient relationship with the author or publisher. The reader must seek the services of a qualified professional for such advice. The author and publisher cannot be held responsible for any financial or health care decisions made by the reader. The author and publisher make no warranty with respect to the completeness or accuracy of the contents of the book, and disclaim any responsibility for any liability, loss, or risk, personal or otherwise, which is incurred as a consequence of the use or application. All coupons, rebates, and other incentives cited are subject to change without notice.

While the author has made every effort to provide accurate telephone numbers and Internet addresses at the time of publication, neither the publisher nor the author assumes any responsibility for errors, or for changes that occur after publication. Further, the publisher does not have any control over and does not assume any responsibility for author or third-party Web sites or their content.

This book is dedicated to the Smile Train,
Changing the World One Smile at a Time,
and to all Americans seeking the path
to affordable health care.

Contents

Chapter Three. Save Money on Preventive Health Care   45

Chapter Four. Save Money on Chronic Health Problems   69

Acknowledgments

Though this book popped into my head seemingly overnight, it was years in the making. If all my patients had been affluent and well insured, I wouldn't have twenty years of experience looking for ways to help them save money. Their questions and needs provided the basis for this work. Additionally, the daily exercise of interpreting the medical world for them in layman's terms smoothed the way to explaining these same concepts to a wider audience. I am indebted to my patients for sharing their trials and triumphs with me, and for teaching me what it takes to be a good doctor.

I am indebted to my colleagues as well. My appreciation goes out to everyone in the community of healers who has contributed to the learning process through books, journals, Web sites, lectures, and personal instruction. Speaking on behalf of doctors today, I thank earlier generations of physicians who pioneered the way.

A special thanks to the American Academy of Family Physicians for their ongoing efforts in promoting primary care medicine in these challenging economic times. I have been a member of the AAFP since first passing my boards in 1986. The opportunities they afford for continuing medical education are unequaled, and their dedication to providing America with quality family physicians is unsurpassed.

Whereas pharmaceutical companies are often condemned for high prices and high profits, I am grateful that they paved the way to the affordable medications we enjoy today. My thanks to the pharmaceutical representatives whom I engaged in friendly banter about the cost of their products. Thanks for the information you share and for helping patients across America with samples, coupons, and rebates.

Physicians cannot provide the help we do without the assistance of dedicated support staff. Thank you, Sandy, for keeping everything organized during the days I spent writing, for always being kind to our patients, and for reminding me to take my cell phone home.

This updated edition of *101 Ways to Save Money on Health Care* would not have been possible without the efforts of Becky Cole, senior editor at Plume, who saw the need to bring this message to a wider audience, and of Nadia Kashper, who served as editor in Becky's absence. Thanks to everyone at Penguin for helping Americans and America a step further along the path to affordable health care.

My gratitude to Terrie Wolf at AKA Literary for her friendship and assistance in navigating the publishing world, and to Neil Erickson for opening my eyes to greater possibilities. May this mark the beginning of a long and propitious relationship.

On a personal note, thank you, Mom, for always being there, and for your endless support, page after page after page. And thank you, Katrina Marie, for your enthusiasm and artistic input. Thank you, K. D. and Luke, for your forbearance, as the laundry piled skyward and cooking became a lost art. Thank you, Celeste and Adam, for being too healthy to need this book. And how could I forget my goldendoodles, Labor and Waffles, who insisted I not sit at my computer all day and helped me maintain a sense of humor throughout this writing experience? I love you all.

And last, but most important, eternal thanks to my Creator for setting me on my journey, and for His daily love and guidance.

Introduction

One year ago I awoke with no special goal in mind. By evening I had a message to take to the world.

It started as an ordinary day. I put the dogs out, took my son to school, spent the day seeing patients, made dinner (this was back in the days when I cooked), cleaned up, and sat down to watch television with my son.

Though he's a teenager, my son likes politics. Together we had watched the presidential campaign and debates about health reform.

Like many health professionals, I was skeptical. But with the 2008 election a done deal, I wanted to give our new leaders a chance. Perhaps it was possible to effect change. Perhaps with years of serious analysis our health care system could be mended.

I was only half listening when I heard the words: health reform by August.

What did he say? Did I hear right? I wondered, leaning forward.

Health reform in six months? I couldn't believe my ears.

No way could the job be accomplished in that short a period. Surely our new administration would take its time, consider the problem carefully, solicit input from medical experts with years of hands-on experience.

Six months? That's when I realized it was politics, not health reform. Politicians couldn't save my patients money. How could they? They were in the business of spending tax-payer money, not saving it. In fact, the statement made me angry.

I bet I know a hundred ways to save money on health care right now, I said to myself. Grabbing a pencil and a piece of notebook paper, I sat down at the kitchen table and started scribbling. Half an hour later the task was complete.

I almost threw that list away. I'd had my catharsis. But then I started thinking: these ideas could help a lot of people—not just my patients. As a physician I understood the system in a way patients did not. Why not share this insider information with the world? Why not turn the list into a book?

I decided to self-publish to get the word out quickly, before the six months were up. I decided to write a page a day. By 100 days I was done, or so I thought. In reality, I'd just begun.

I wasn't alone in looking for an answer to help Americans save on health care. While I was busy with my book in Ohio, a thoughtful editor in New York was working along the same lines. Though I lacked the means to share my message across America, Plume, an imprint of Penguin, was well equipped to do so. The book you are reading is a collaborative update of the original self-published work.

As Americans we like to be in charge of our own destiny.

But when it comes to health care, we often feel powerless. We have little way of determining the true cost. We don't understand our options and are frequently afraid to ask.

And the expense can be overwhelming. According to the 2009 Milliman Medical Index, the medical cost for a typical American family of four was $16,771, including insurance cost, per year. Of this, $9,947 was paid by the employer, with the remainder made up by $4,004 in employee contributions and $2,820 in out-of-pocket expenditures. But that $9,947 from your employer's pocket, isn't it really your own?

Overall, uninsured patients spend only half as much out of pocket as insured patients—but why? Those who are young and healthy hope to save money by avoiding the expense of insurance. That works fine, until you break a bone or contract appendicitis. Other patients simply cannot afford health care, let alone health insurance. When uninsured medical expenses reach thousands of dollars, many patients simply cannot pay—amounting to over $50,000,000,000 in uncompensated care in 2008.

Insured and uninsured patients alike dread the possibility of serious illness. It's bad enough to be gravely sick or injured without having to worry about losing your home, your car, or your job. What if you develop cancer or require dialysis? Will insurance cover the hundreds of thousands of dollars such care will cost? Will you be forced to go on welfare?

As a physician I've seen patients struggle with the choice of health care or house payments. Even as a doctor I've been faced with rationing my family's health care: do we spend thousands of dollars out of pocket for dental care or use that money for college tuition?

In recent months the national debate on health reform has added to the aura of uncertainty. It's possible that health care reform will cost Americans even more. Is there some way the nation can provide better health care to every citizen without increasing the tax burden? Where are the hidden costs?

The more I listened to the debate, the more I felt it was my duty as a physician to help people stay healthy *and* save money today—not ten years from now. I decided to become an advocate, to share "tricks of the trade" that physicians know, but of which patients may be unaware. I wanted to put a tool in the hands of the individual to help people regain control over their finances and their future.

Of course, the best way to save money on health care is not to need it in the first place. Take care of yourself, eat healthy, exercise daily, stop smoking, lose weight, and avoid self-destructive behavior.

But beyond that, this book offers you an insider's look at health care costs and how to save. As a family physician I don't have all the answers for high-ticket items, like a heart bypass or bone marrow transplant. But I do have a good understanding of how the average American can save money—real money—on health care expenses.

In this book you'll find ways to save money on doctor visits, prescription medications, preventive health care, and chronic disease. You'll learn how you can limit your out-of-pocket expenses for acute illness, medical testing, hospital bills, and ancillary health services. And you'll find dozens of ways to treat yourself at home with over-the-counter remedies and nonprescription medications.

These opportunities to save are organized in ten chapters, one on each of the above topics, with ten money-saving tips included in each chapter. Chapter 11 offers a summary with advice for thinking ahead. If you don't see a topic listed, consult the index.

Pricing mentioned throughout the book is based on information garnered from various sources including current Medicare and insurance reimbursement rates, typical negotiated fee schedules and discounts, and online and retail pharmacy pricing. These prices change quite frequently; they are listed to give you an approximation of those you'll find in your own community.

Unless you *never* need a doctor, you will save money using this consumer guide. With the money you save, won't you consider being a blessing to others?

Since 1999 the Smile Train has helped thousands of children each year who suffer from cleft lip or cleft palate, both in the United States and abroad. For as little as $250 a child can receive this life-changing surgery. Donate online today at www.smiletrain.org and help change the world, one smile at a time. A portion of the author's proceeds from this book will be donated to the Smile Train.

Health and happiness to you and yours,

CYNTHIA J. KOELKER, MD

101 Ways to
Save Money
on Health Care

CHAPTER ONE

Save Money on Doctor Visits

1. Avoid unnecessary doctor visits

The first way to save money at the doctor is: don't go when you don't need to.

But how's a person to know? Sadly, there is no simple answer. The decision involves a degree of common sense, life experience, and medical knowledge.

If you think you may need to see a doctor, ask someone you trust first. Ask your mother, ask your grandmother, ask the lady down the street who has raised a dozen kids. Try the local ask-a-nurse hotline.

Many hospitals offer a free ask-a-nurse hotline as a medical triage service to their communities. Do an online search for your locale, or call your local hospital or medical society for further information. If you request their ask-a-nurse hotline, they'll know what you mean. The hotlines are generally staffed with registered nurses, who follow standard protocols in answering your questions. They are especially helpful in determining if your situation requires immediate medical attention.

Or call your trusted family doctor. When you call, give an accurate but brief synopsis of your problem. Include your symptoms, how long you've had them, how bad they are, and whether they're changing. Ask the doctor (or her nurse) if you should be seen or if you should give your body more time to heal on its own. If they determine no appointment is necessary, ask for a time frame—how long to wait and what to watch for.

Head colds are probably the number one reason patients make unnecessary doctor visits. Keep in mind a typical head cold resolves in a week without treatment—or seven days with treatment. Most people suffering from head cold symptoms can wait it out.

Antibiotics don't help a cold virus anyway—your own immune system heals you. But when symptoms progressively worsen or go into your chest, then a visit to your physician is warranted.

In general, doctors would rather treat someone who truly needs medical attention than offer treatment (or worse yet, antibiotics) to a patient simply to justify the time and expense involved with an office visit. Chicken soup is cheaper than ciprofloxacin.

Many minor accidents and illnesses may be treated at home—where to draw the line is the question. Here are a few guidelines to help you decide whether to see your doctor:

- Minor sprains usually resolve within a few days. If rest, ice, compression (an elastic bandage), and elevation don't relieve your symptoms (acronym: RICE), see your doctor.

- Likewise, back pain in a weekend warrior should abate with rest, heat or ice, over-the-counter NSAIDs (see #96), and avoidance of heavy lifting or strain.
- Burns that don't cause blistering just need to be kept clean and free from reinjury.
- Bee stings that swell only at the site of the sting (without symptoms elsewhere, such as hives or trouble breathing) can be treated with over-the-counter oral antihistamines (see #97).
- Lastly, a broken heart often responds to a hot fudge sundae.
- If in doubt, call first.

2. Partner with your doctor

Does your doctor know who you are? If not, you haven't established an effective partnership.

I know I just said to avoid unnecessary visits. But if your doctor doesn't remember who you are, odds are he or she won't help you without first seeing you.

Every day, doctors assist patients without charging them, from refills to phone advice or return-to-work forms. If your doctor doesn't know you, these courtesies will not be available to you.

Most doctors consider a year since your last visit as the outside limit for when they might offer phone advice or perhaps refill a medication without an appointment first—and *that's* assuming they know you and trust you. If you haven't seen your doctor for the last three years, you would be considered a new patient according to Current Procedural Terminology (CPT) coding.

Even if you're rarely ill, it would be a good idea to see your family doctor once a year. Don't feel bad about going when nothing's wrong—physicians would love to hear you say, "I'm not really sick; I just want you to know who I am in case I ever need you." Such an appointment could be used to discuss updating vaccines, routine screening tests, or perhaps that nagging itch you wouldn't bother to seek medical attention for otherwise. The visit may last only a few minutes and may cost considerably less than a longer visit for an illness.

Patients who see their physicians on a regular basis would benefit from effective partnering as well. Do you call your doctor more than once between visits? Whereas an occasional phone call is reasonable and often advisable, repeat calls suggest that you may benefit from spacing your office visits closer together in order to address additional concerns (see #5 and #6).

If you have multiple problems (such as diabetes, high blood pressure, high cholesterol, and migraines), it is not reasonable to expect they can all be thoroughly addressed in a single ten-minute visit. In most offices longer appointments are available, but you'll need to request the extra time when you schedule your upcoming visit. Otherwise, either your concerns will remain unmet, or spending extra time with you will make your doctor run late, causing frustration among staff and patients alike.

Longer office visits cost more than shorter visits but are still less expensive than multiple appointments. For insured patients they offer the advantage of saving a second co-pay.

Ask the receptionist how much a longer visit will cost and how much time the doctor is likely to spend with you. This should help you decide what best suits your needs. Sometimes shorter, more frequent appointments are the way to go, since longer visits can become too complex for a patient to absorb at one sitting, even with note-taking.

If you do decide you'd like a longer appointment and understand the cost implications, don't forget to tell the receptionist when you schedule your visit. Otherwise, you'll be given a standard ten-minute slot, which may be insufficient to address your needs. If you don't mind having another person in the room, bring along a friend or family member. Two sets of ears are better than one.

3. See your family doctor, not a specialist

Did you know consultants charge more, often considerably more, for what is commonly the same service your family doctor might render?

If you need a heart bypass or perhaps a hysterectomy, by all means, see a specialist. But if you have a common malady such as acne, asthma, or anxiety, your family physician is well equipped to diagnose and treat these conditions. And odds are, you'll save money.

Not only is your family physician (or other primary care physician) likely to charge you less, family doctors are less likely to order expensive testing. Specialists often look for a definitive diagnosis, whereas your family doctor may focus more on symptom relief. He or she may offer a therapeutic trial of medicine, reserving costly testing for conditions that aren't easily resolved.

Family doctors aren't just for colds and sore throats. They're trained to handle 90 to 95 percent of conditions encountered in their daily practice. This list of conditions is long and overlaps considerably with a broad range of subspecialties.

If you have a problem and wonder whether your doctor can address it, give her a call. If she cannot, she'll refer you to a trusted specialist, ideally one she'd be willing to see herself.

Below is a noninclusive list of conditions and services, from head to toe, that family doctors treat or offer on a daily basis, ones for which, under most circumstances, a specialty consult is not required.

- Acne, psoriasis, eczema, headache, migraine, insomnia, anxiety, depression, Alzheimer's disease, rosacea, stress
- Ear infection, hearing loss, dizziness
- Pink eye, styes, scleral hemorrhage
- Allergies, sinusitis, nose bleed
- Mouth ulcers, thrush, tonsillitis, parotiditis
- Swollen glands, goiter, stiff neck
- Asthma, chronic obstructive pulmonary disease (COPD), emphysema, laryngitis, bronchitis, pneumonia
- Stable heart failure, stable angina, chronic atrial fibrillation, most heart murmurs, most palpitations, most chest pain

- Acid reflux, ulcers, indigestion, diarrhea, constipation, irritable bowel syndrome, diverticulitis, hemorrhoids
- Urine infections, kidney stones, overactive bladder, incontinence, prostate infection or benign prostatic enlargement
- Pap smears, birth control, menopause, menstrual cramping or irregularity
- Diabetes, thyroid disease, weight loss or gain, obesity
- Back pain, sciatica, carpal tunnel syndrome, arthritis, warts, nail fungus

---

One Bit of Good News for Medicare Patients (but Bad News for Specialists)

Traditionally specialists have been paid higher fees by using so-called "consultation codes." As of 2010 Medicare no longer allows the distinction between regular office visit codes and consultation codes. For the time being, consultation codes are still permitted for privately insured patients.

Though family doctors will be little affected, specialists may suffer a significant drop in income. Were it not for the vociferous health care debate, this coding change would have spurred a huge outcry from specialists. It remains to be seen whether the change will benefit patients directly. Though the reimbursement for Medicare patients will be lower, access to care may be compromised, leading to no net gain—another reason to see your family physician if at all possible.

4. See the right eye doctor for you

True or false? All eye doctors are created equal.

Most people think of an eye doctor as the person who examines their eyes in order to obtain glasses.

Strictly speaking, an eye doctor is an ophthalmologist, a physician trained in the diagnosis and treatment of diseases of the eye, including cataracts, glaucoma, or problems resulting from diabetes or high blood pressure. Ophthalmologists prescribe eye medications and perform eye surgery, but often prescribe eyeglasses or contacts as well.

An optometrist, also commonly referred to as an eye doctor, is not a physician, but rather a trained professional licensed to examine patients for visual defects, and to prescribe glasses and contact lenses. The glasses themselves are made by an optician.

An optometrist usually offers a lower examination fee than an ophthalmologist. If you're healthy, have no insurance, and only need a pair of glasses, see your local optometrist (or the one employed at your local superstore).

If you have insurance, check your policy to decide what type of eye doctor to see. If your coverage offers an annual eye exam, most likely this is through an optometrist on your plan.

If, however, you have a medical problem, it may cost you less to see an ophthalmologist. Ophthalmologists are covered under your insurance (including Medicare) the same as any other specialist, such as a cardiologist. (Traditional Medicare does not cover optometrists, though it is possible your secondary insurance may pay.) Any person with high blood pressure or diabetes has a valid reason to see an ophthalmologist.

Physicians and optometrists both refer patients to ophthalmologists for a variety of conditions including certain infections, injuries to the eye, uncorrectable visual problems, lazy eyes, glaucoma, cataracts, persistent styes, macular degeneration, diabetic or hypertensive retinopathy, iritis, and droopy eyelids.

Prescription eye medications are covered under both insurance and Medicare the same as any other prescription medication. Medicare does not pay for routine vision testing, eyeglasses, or contact lenses. They do cover "standard frames" after cataract surgery, although patients may choose to pay the difference for an upgrade to a "deluxe frame" of their own choosing.

Even if you have no disease of the eye other than poor vision, your insurance may cover a visit to a medical eye doctor. Again, check your policy first for coverage and your list of in-network physicians (ophthalmologists), optometrists, and opticians.

5. Plan ahead and combine visits

One longer visit with your doctor is almost always cheaper than two shorter visits.

The immediate savings for insured patients is obvious, with only one co-payment due rather than two. But even for self-pay patients, longer visits are often more cost-effective.

But my doctor will only see me for one problem at a time,

you say. The reasons for this are likely rooted in a combination of coding and scheduling. If you take the time to a) understand the system and b) work with the person in charge of appointment scheduling, you'll find your doctor more willing to accommodate you.

Doctors submit CPT (Current Procedural Terminology) codes to insurance companies (and Medicare) in order to get paid. These codes focus on the complexity of a *single* problem rather than the *number* of problems treated at a given visit. Current CPT coding works well for specialists, who generally treat one organ system, such as the heart. But the system does not work well for primary care physicians, who may treat the same patient for diabetes, hypertension, high cholesterol, asthma, and warts all on the same day.

Three straightforward problems could easily take more time than a single complex problem, yet the codes were not designed to reflect this. Therefore, many doctors have chosen to limit patients to one problem per office visit.

Yet it is perfectly reasonable for patients to hope their physician would treat them for an acute problem at the time of a previously scheduled visit for a chronic illness such as diabetes or depression.

Also, doctors don't like to be surprised by extra problems, nor do they enjoy trying to do the work of two problems in the time allotted to one. And believe me, *it happens every day*.

How to resolve the dilemma? The solution lies in planning ahead. (In the long run, doctors hope for a change in the system of coding as well.) An appointment for a blood pressure check could be combined with a visit for bronchitis, but you need to call beforehand, explain the situation, and request more time. If a longer appointment is not available at the original appointment time, ask for a different time or different day.

Your doctor will want to allow sufficient time to address your multiple concerns adequately. Calling ahead alerts the office staff to the need for special coding (modifiers) when a procedure (such as an ear irrigation or wart freezing) is combined with an E&M (evaluation & management) service.

A Pap smear or breast exam might be combined with a routine visit for, say, headaches. A follow-up on depression could be combined with a flare-up of allergies.

The list is endless but the point is clear. *Two problems take longer than one, but one visit is cheaper than two.* Plan ahead and your doctor will work with you for a happier solution.

One Thing Patients Should Know

When doctors combine visits, or do two procedures at the same office visit, they generally make less money than if the procedures or visits were scheduled on separate days. Whereas this makes the patient happy, it doesn't necessarily please the doctor.

My focus here is helping you, the patient, save money on health care (with an apology to the doctors). Remember, though, that for every $50 you save, your doctor loses $50. So at least send a thank-you card. Doctors are human, too. Their hearts are warmed when their good deeds are appreciated. It's not all about the money.

6. Organize your thoughts

Why are you seeing your doctor? You'd be surprised how often a patient doesn't know.

Before you step foot in your doctor's office, ask yourself, *Why am I going?* If you know why you're going, what you want to accomplish, and prepare accordingly, you'll derive significantly greater benefit from your visit and save money as well.

Husbands are notorious for not knowing why they've come. *The wife sent me*, they say, not really wanting to be there at all. Older people are unclear as to the exact reason for visits as well. *I'm here for a checkup*, they respond, expecting the doctor to discover anything that may be ailing them. *I need my pills*, others may answer, knowing neither the name nor purpose of their medications. Figuring out why a person has come to the doctor often takes more time than deciding proper treatment.

Save money by saving time. Though charges for physician visits are not based solely on time spent with a patient, it does factor into the equation. Remember, time is money, and someone is keeping track. Many physicians note the time they enter a patient's room and the time they leave, for billing purposes. You can save money by doing the same. Time flies when you're the center of attention. It may seem only ten minutes have passed when it's been half an hour. Keep track and stay focused.

Know if you're due for blood work—if you don't come in fasting, you may need to return, perhaps missing another hour of work (and income). Have a urine problem? Bring a fresh, refrigerated specimen in a clean glass jar. Have a knee problem? Wear shorts or a skirt to hasten the exam. Bad toe? Take off your socks and shoes—do you really want to pay the doctor to watch you do so? Need refills? Check your prescriptions before you leave home. Make a list of what you have and what you'll need for your doctor to review.

Much can be accomplished if your goals are clear. Get a notebook and jot down your thoughts. Make a list of what you hope to address. But please don't make a "shopping list" of twenty items. Neither you nor your doctor can focus adequately on more than a few problems at a time, usually not more than two or three. Prioritize your needs and let your doctor know what concerns you most. Ask your doctor how many of them can be addressed in one visit. Ask if you should make a second appointment to address the others and if so, how soon. After your visit, make additional notes regarding your doctor's comments and plans.

A little-advertised truth is that what a doctor charges has an element of flexibility to it. The same work might be accomplished in fifteen minutes or half an hour, depending on several factors, some of which are within your control. Your doctor is more likely to throw in a "freebie" if you make your requests known up front and stay on task. But if you wait until your doctor is about to leave the room to ask about a second problem, he or she will groan inwardly (if not audibly) and may adjust your bill upward.

Stay focused, save time, and you'll save money. Ask your doctor if this isn't true.

7. Lengthen the interval between visits

My sessions often end with a patient asking me, *When do you want to see me again?* My answer is, *It depends.*

It depends on your age, your condition, your understanding of your medical problems, and often your compliance with the therapeutic plan. And it may depend on your finances. A better question might be *why* you should return at a particular time.

Both you and your doctor share the responsibility for your health care. If your doctor trusts you, he or she will gladly relinquish much of your care to you, the patient.

For this to work, however, you must do your part. For example, doctors don't want to be held responsible for patients who take their medicines incorrectly. If a diabetic (who knows better) doesn't take his insulin correctly, his blood sugar will be too high or too low. He may end up in a coma—or worse. No doctor can help a patient who won't help himself. For good reason doctors require less reliable patients to be seen more frequently.

But if you and your doctor share an understanding of your treatment, your doctor will trust you to return less often. For the same condition, one patient is examined monthly, another might be seen every three months, and another perhaps every six. The difference? The patient's condition and his or her compliance, understanding, age, memory, and occasionally finances.

Doctors are more likely to trust patients who:

- Show up for their appointments
- Know their medications
- Understand their condition or illness
- Take care of themselves

Using diabetes as an example again, if you control your blood sugar, along with your cholesterol and blood pressure, the interval between visits might be stretched from, say, three months to four months, saving you the cost of one office visit and one set of blood work per year, easily over $100. The same applies to other chronic illnesses/conditions such as asthma, depression, and high blood pressure.

The point here is to take control of your health care, not to compromise it. Be responsible and your doctor will trust you to come less frequently.

8. If possible, avoid urgent visits

Why do urgent visits cost more? In a word, *coding.*

Doctors normally charge according to a book of Current Procedural Terminology (CPT) codes, which lists every procedure from splinter removal to splenectomy.

There are codes for *routine* procedures or office visits, and codes for *emergency* (or *urgent*) visits. Extra time and urgent visits cost more.

An urgent visit might be one where you show up at the doctor's office without calling first. Some doctors code urgent visits whenever a patient calls to be seen *the same day* for, say, a bad cough. Although many doctors do not "code higher" for a same-day appointment, they do have the right to do so—and to charge more. After all, if the doctor did not accommodate your need, you might end up at the emergency room—which costs *much* more.

What a patient considers urgent likely differs from a doctor's opinion. Although some patients wait too long to seek medical care, it is more common for a patient to believe he needs urgent attention when his problem could easily have waited a day or two (see #1).

If you think you need urgent attention (and don't have an experienced adult to tell you otherwise), call your doctor and ask.

Ask specifically if you need to be seen right away or if your problem can wait for a nonurgent appointment. Ask what you should do in the meantime to alleviate the symptoms. Ask about anything that would alert you to the need for an emergency room visit.

A good number of the problems that present urgently to a doctor's office resolve on their own within a few days. Most sprained ankles don't need immediate attention—if you can walk, odds are it isn't broken (see #47).

The idea is not to put your health at risk but rather to allow your body to heal on its own. Other problems of potentially nonurgent nature include:

- **Sore throats:** Unless you're deathly ill, a sore throat can wait a few days—even if it's strep. If your throat is so swollen you can't breathe, if you have a serious underlying condition such as rheumatic heart disease, or if you're so sick you can't get out of bed, by all means, seek medical attention immediately.

• **Ear infections:** We all have sympathy for a child crying with ear pain, but what is needed is pain relief, not antibiotics. Using a hot water bottle to warm the ear often helps significantly, as does Tylenol or ibuprofen. If these measures relieve the pain, waiting a few days to see a doctor is reasonable.

• **Fever:** The best way to gauge whether you need to see a doctor is how sick you are otherwise. If you or your child is not especially ill—still up and about, playing and eating—give it a few days. Unless a fever is quite high (say above 104 degrees Fahrenheit), there is no need (other than comfort) to lower one's temperature. The severity of symptoms other than fever should determine whether you should seek medical care.

• **Stomach flu or diarrhea:** The biggest risk is dehydration, which takes at least a few days to develop in an adult, though may occur more quickly in a small child. Again, the biggest question is how sick you are overall. If you're not too ill—not dizzy, overly weak, or in pain—wait a few days.

• **Head colds and sinus infections:** If it's just a cold, wait a good week before consulting a doctor. If you have asthma, COPD, a history of pneumonia, unstable diabetes, cancer, or other serious illness, you should have already developed a contingency plan with your doctor's input. If not, see your doctor if you're not improving within a few days.

- **Sprains where you still have use of the affected limb:** Rest, Ice, Compression, Elevation (RICE) are the mainstays of treatment. Your symptoms should be at their worst by 48 hours after injury, then begin resolving. If this isn't the case, see your doctor.

- **Insect bite/sting with local symptoms only:** Usually localized pain and swelling resolve the same day, or the next, or the next. Do what doctors do: outline the area of redness or swelling using a ballpoint pen, to better determine whether the area is enlarging. If it's not, and if no other symptoms occur, waiting several days is fine. If the area is expanding or becoming more painful, see your doctor.

If in doubt, call your doctor. Ask whether you need to be seen the same day. Ask whether there is an extra charge for urgent visits. Ask whether the problem can wait a day or two, especially if she's too busy to see you. Perhaps you'll be well in a day or two, and won't need to be seen at all.

9. Ask to pay by the hour

As I said before, time is money, and someone's keeping track.

At least for self-paying patients, it's *your* time and *your* money, so *you* should be the one with the stopwatch.

In order to stay on schedule and for billing purposes, I document the time I enter each patient room and the time I leave. Patients are often surprised when I say it's been a half hour and I need to move on. To them it seemed much shorter. Most patients aren't counting their time the same way medical offices do, and many don't understand that longer office visits cost more.

You could save money by contracting with your doctor for a certain amount of time. The impetus will be up to you rather than the doctor to complete your business in a timely fashion, but you should be able to do this if you organize your thoughts ahead of time. Some doctors contract for services on a minute by minute basis, though that makes it difficult to predict what the final bill will be. I suggest asking your doctor how much she would charge for a visit lasting 10, 15, 20, 30, 45, or 60 minutes *if you pay in cash ahead of time*.

If you don't intend to pay at the time of the visit, it's unlikely your doctor will accept your proposal. Billing is expensive and human nature is fickle. Every doctor's been burned by someone who's promised to pay but didn't.

Contracting for time bypasses the coding and billing system doctors normally employ. Such visits cannot be submitted for insurance reimbursement. If your doctor is a Medicare provider, he or she cannot contract for time for services normally covered under Medicare but is permitted do so for services not covered, such as certain preventive services or cosmetic procedures. Your doctor is more likely to consider contracting for time for evaluation and management services than for procedural services with additional overhead, such as minor surgery.

Contracting for time may be useful when you have multiple problems that you'd like to get handled on the same day, or when two or three family members are ill at the same time. Doctors don't like to feel pressured to cram two patients or two problems into the time allotted for one—neither ends up getting the proper attention. But look how relaxed your doctor appears when you pay him ahead of time for 30 or 60 minutes of medical care! Suddenly, the onus is on you to have your thoughts organized. *You'll* be the one wanting to get more accomplished in a given amount of time. *You'll* be the one wanting to leave the room first.

To get the full benefit of this approach, plan ahead, organize your thoughts, check if you need refills, review your formulary (see #11), bring a record of your blood sugar or blood pressure, fill out your portion of any forms you need to have completed, get a copy of the "$4 list" (see #16) from your local pharmacy, and keep a notebook with questions and notes from previous visits.

Make a computer file of your medicines and print an updated list for every visit. Bring two copies of an organized, detailed description of your problems, leaving room for your doctor's comments and your own. If you contract for time for multiple family members, make separate lists for each person's individual chart.

Your doctor will appreciate your preparedness, and your efficiency will be a breath of fresh air.

10. Ask your doctor for a discount

With fear and trembling, I suggest you ask your doctor for a discount. From across the nation, I hear the thunder of doctors' feathers ruffling.

But aren't all doctors rich, you might ask?

A primary care physician (PCP) working full-time (50-plus hours per week) earns the equivalent of a middle-aged couple, both employed as public school teachers. Are teachers rich? Few would say so. (Specialists may make two to four times as much as primary care physicians, fueling class envy even among the professionals.)

But back to your family doc. Overall, we're a compassionate group. We became doctors to help people, after all. And given the right circumstances, most would consider granting a discount.

Before you ask, however, here are a few things to keep in mind.

First, your doctor may have already discounted her fee without you even asking. Perhaps she's charged you for only ten minutes of her time when you've taken thirty. The receptionist may be able to tell you if this is so, or could apprise you of your doctor's usual and customary charges.

Second, be reasonable. If you spend $100 a month on cigarettes or alcohol or lottery tickets, is it fair to ask your doctor to subsidize your habit?

Third, a word about co-pays. Your doctor is required by law and contract to collect these payments. Under most co-pay situations the fee has already been "adjusted" downward by 30, 40, or even 50 percent. If a doctor charges you, say, $100, insurance often knocks that down to about $65, the remaining $35 simply disappearing as a "negotiated" adjustment. Of the remaining $65 a good $40 goes to overhead (staff, malpractice, rent, utilities, equipment, etc.).

If your insurance pays $40 of the $65 "negotiated fee," that leaves your $25 co-pay to cover the doctor's time with you. These "negotiated fees" have dropped so low that many doctors are finding it difficult to stay in business.

If you have financial concerns, talk to your doctor about a discount. For obvious reasons self-pay patients have a vested interest in this option. Don't assume your doctor knows your financial situation. Speak up.

Depending on the office setup, the best person to ask could be your doctor, her office manager, or the billing department. It may also depend on whether your doctor is self-employed or an employee. In a large medical office there may be policies in place for dealing with discount requests. Bills generated by doctors who are hospital employees may be eligible for discounts under the same guidelines that hospitals use (see #54 and #64). Sometimes it's easier to request a discount at these large facilities where policies are impersonal.

If you see a doctor in a small office, ask the doctor directly. If you're embarrassed to do that, ask the receptionist or nurse, who will then ask the doctor for you.

Consider ahead of time what is fair. If your doctor writes off your entire bill, he is actually losing money every time he sees you—no doubt his office staff still wants to get paid, along with the utility company and mortgage holder. Paying half a doctor's charges at least allows your doctor to cover his overhead, though he himself will be working for free.

If you need a discount, I suggest you ask for up to a third off your bill, bringing it down to the amount Medicare would pay. If your request is granted, send a note or bring a pie. You'll feel good about it and so will your doctor.

But if you're stuck in a terrible situation beyond your

control, your doctor might see you for free. Again it's a matter of trust—trust that you're doing what you can to help yourself.

Here are some other options:

• Self-pay patients should consider asking for a billing discount for cash up front (meaning, you pay in full at the time of service, negating the need for the office to bill you in the future). A billing discount may be as little as $5 or $10, but that's still enough for a meal.

• Many medical offices allow interest-free monthly payments. Set up a payment schedule and stick to it. Don't just disappear without a word.

• If there's any way you can pay ahead a little, send your doctor $20 a month, prepaid. That's less than a dollar a day—almost anyone could afford that. Then when you need medical care, you'll have a credit to draw from, and you can still ask for a discount, a request your doctor is much more likely to grant since you've shown an amazing degree of responsibility.

• Barter is another option if you have services to trade. You'll never know unless you ask. Have a small business? Treat your doctor well—he or she will remember you and return the kindness. And lastly, some doctors still accept payment in chickens.

CHAPTER TWO

Save Money on Prescription Medications

11. Know your formulary

If you have prescription coverage, odds are you have a formulary, whether you know it or not.

Most insurance companies maintain formularies, or lists of drugs that they pay for as a plan benefit, usually using a tiered system. Less expensive drugs have the lowest co-pay (Tier 1), the most expensive drugs have the highest co-pay (Tier 3), and the remainder lie in between (Tier 2). This tier designation does not go strictly on retail price—insurance companies negotiate with pharmaceutical companies for discounts that in some instances may make a costlier drug preferred over a less costly one.

Formularies are organized along therapeutic classes. For example, they all contain several blood pressure pills, antibiotics, and diabetic medications. Within each major therapeutic class are various subclasses. Your formulary is unlikely to include more than one or two medications from each subclass, especially when only brand-name products are available. For example, subclasses for the treatment of high blood pressure include beta-blockers, alpha-blockers, diuretics, calcium channel blockers, ACE inhibitors, and angiotensin receptor blockers. Prior to 2010 the angiotensin receptor blockers were brand name only. It is likely your formulary includes only one or two of the several that are available, and each formulary is different. As drug patents expire and generics become available, your formulary is likely to change. If your doctor chooses from your list, it will save you money.

How does your doctor know what to choose? Chances are, she doesn't, not unless she has access to your formulary. Get two copies—bring one with you to every doctor visit. Have your doctor keep the other in your chart for reference.

Keep in mind, however, that Tier 1 drugs may not necessarily be your first choice. You may be intolerant of a certain drug, or perhaps unresponsive to it. You may have been stable on a particular name-brand prescription for years already and are therefore hesitant to make a change. Some medications require blood-level monitoring, and levels may be more consistent with brand-name medications, so switching to a generic may not save you money if you need to have your blood level checked more often.

Additional savings are available in the form of coupons or rebates (see #12) from pharmaceutical companies, which may save you $20 to $50 off your co-pay, thereby lowering your out-of-pocket cost for a higher-tiered drug to the same as that of a lower-tiered medication. One reason retail drug prices have increased in recent years is so the pharmaceutical companies can offer these discounts, thus making their brand-name products more competitive with generics.

Know your formulary—and partner with your doctor to save you money.

12. Look for coupons

Would you clip a coupon to save 10¢ on a can of beans? Much greater savings are available using coupons for brand-name prescription medications.

Pharmaceutical companies offer coupons for discounts or rebates for two reasons: to encourage you to try their medication, or to keep you on it.

Coupons are available through your doctor, your pharmacist, or online. You may also find offers in your local newspaper or favorite magazine.

Some pharmaceutical companies offer coupons for a free trial of medication, from a three-day introductory offer to an entire month's prescription free. Others offer a discount or rebate on your out-of-pocket expense, including co-pay amounts, as high as $55 a month. Some are one-time offers, but many are renewable for a few months, or a year, or even for as long as you require the medication. The reusable coupons usually come in the form of a card that you present to the pharmacy each time you need a refill. If the discount is in the form of a rebate, make sure you keep your receipts.

If you are already on medication, or if your doctor prescribes a new medication, ask if it is name brand. If so, ask whether your doctor has a coupon. Since this takes an extra minute or so, your doctor may not remember to offer. If you forget to ask the doctor, ask the nurse or receptionist. If your doctor does not have a coupon that does not mean one isn't available. Many doctors are too busy to talk with pharmaceutical representatives, who are the primary source of these coupons. Your next step is to either ask the pharmacist or check online. Sometimes the coupons a doctor or pharmacist has available offer a better discount than what can be found online. Other times the offers are identical.

Start an online search by entering "drug name" and "coupon," but beware as some offers may be from illegitimate sites. Look for the pharmaceutical company's Web site or the domain name for the medication, then look for special offers. Sometimes you can print a coupon straight off a Web page. Other times you must first submit personal identifying information.

Some of these programs are not available to government-sponsored (Medicare and Medicaid) prescription-plan beneficiaries. Read the fine print or ask your pharmacist.

A second type of coupon is offered through retail pharmacies and commonly involves new or transfer prescriptions. The coupon may be worth more than the price of the drug you are purchasing. Some stores will honor another retailer's coupon as well. Theoretically, you could actually make a profit—transfer a $5 prescription and receive $20 in store merchandise. Stores do this to get you in the door, hoping you'll become a repeat customer or buy additional products.

Retail pharmacy coupons may appear in local publications, or show up in your personal mail. In general, they apply to either generic or brand-name medications. Discounts may be offered on current or future prescriptions, other store merchandise, or even gasoline purchases. Some retailers offer gift cards rather than discounts. Large retailers offer coupons and discounts online as well. Visit your local pharmacy's Web site for additional information.

If you're lucky, you may be able to combine a retail pharmacy coupon with that of a pharmaceutical company. Happy hunting!

13. Ask about price matching

Ever notice how when one gas station lowers its price, the competing station across the street does as well?

Retail pharmacies follow the same practice. In recent years the $4 list has become a prime example of competitive pricing (see #16). Shortly after one discount chain offered a long list of medications for $4 a month, several others followed suit.

Less well known is the unadvertised practice of *price matching*. No retailer wants to lose your business. Just as one megastore may match a competitor's price on a computer printer, so, too, a retail pharmacy may match a competitor's price on penicillin.

But you have to ask. In general retail pharmacies don't advertise this practice. If you shop around and request a quote from a discount chain pharmacy for the price on a particular prescription, your local (perhaps more convenient) pharmacy may well match this lower price.

Retail medication prices include the wholesale cost of the drug, a dispensing fee of a few dollars, and the retail markup.

It is these latter two that allow some leeway in prescription pricing. The retail markup can vary significantly from one pharmacy to another, so it behooves you to check around. A $20 difference in markup is not uncommon. Retail pharmacies offer price matching to generate goodwill among their customers and to keep their business.

Sometimes a pharmacy will price a medication *below* cost (a loss leader) in order to attract additional business to the store, hoping to make a profit on condiments if not medicaments.

But please don't put your local mom-and-pop drugstore out of business. As a solo family physician, I feel the pressure of big medicine on a daily basis. Every mom-and-pop pharmacy in my area has gone out of business or sold out to a chain store. If you ask your independent neighborhood pharmacist for a discount, please also ask how you might support their business in some other way. Buy groceries or school supplies or Band-Aids while you're there. If you value their services, please support them.

14. Consider pill splitting

Splitting pills may not be glamorous, but it could save you big bucks, perhaps hundreds of dollars a year. Many doctors advocate the practice and I've split pills myself. If your doctor is willing to do so, shouldn't you consider pill splitting?

How did this practice originate? Some years ago the pharmaceutical industry introduced the concept of *flat pricing*. Multiple strengths of a given medication are priced the same. (Production cost differs little according to pill strength.) This allows a patient to pay the same amount for a particular drug if the dosage is increased, a cost savings in itself.

The savings increase when flat pricing is combined with pill splitting. For example, if your doctor prescribes 50 milligrams of Drug A, taking half of a (same-priced) 100-milligram pill instead may save you 50 percent off the cost of the medication. *But ask first.* Generally if a pill is scored—if it has a line down the middle to facilitate breaking—it is safe to split. *But always ask your doctor or pharmacist first.*

There are risks of splitting the wrong pills. Cutting time-release tablets may result in an acute overdose, as the entire amount is rapidly absorbed into the bloodstream. Some pills have an enteric coating to protect the stomach lining from the medication. This effect will be lost once the pill has been split.

Common pills that may be safely split include certain cholesterol medications (most statins), certain antidepressants (most SSRIs), many antibiotics, some diabetic medications, and a variety of blood pressure pills.

A pill splitter costs about $5. It holds the pill securely so you can get an accurate split without cutting your fingers. Do not put your fingers inside the razor-sharp pill cutter. *Again, certain pills are dangerous when split, especially time-release medications.*

Pill cutting is not for everyone. Patients with a hand tremor or poor eyesight may lack the dexterity to accomplish the task successfully. If a family member is recruited for the task, make sure the patient understands the intended dosage.

But the average middle-aged American with high cholesterol and kids in college will appreciate the $40 to $400 a year in savings that pill splitting may afford.

I cannot stress this enough: ask your doctor or pharmacist before splitting pills.

15. Save money on brand-name drugs

Is this even possible? Certainly so, even if you have no insurance coverage. But it may take some work on your part.

When your doctor draws out his prescription pad, tell him you'll be paying cash. Ask whether a generic medication would do as well (or nearly so). If he determines a brand-name drug is indicated for your condition, or if no generic is available, ask if there are less expensive choices within the needed therapeutic class. If your doctor doesn't know, have him make two or three suggestions, which you can check at your pharmacy later.

Ask whether the chosen drug has flat pricing and whether your pills may be split. Ask whether you could decrease your dosage or take your medicine less often when your condition is stabilized. This is often possible for asthma or allergy drugs.

Compare prices at several pharmacies. The difference in markup from one pharmacy to another could easily be $20 a month. Then check for pharmaceutical coupons through your doctor, your pharmacy, or online. Next check for coupons from local pharmacies for new or transfer prescriptions (see #12, 13, 14, and 17).

Also ask your pharmacist whether a higher or lower dose of medication would cost less. Commonly used dosage strengths sometimes cost less, even at higher-milligram strength.

Do the Math

The following is an example of what you might save on a brand-name cholesterol drug prescribed when a generic was ineffective or unavailable.

	Cost per year
Pharmacy A List price $150/month	$1800
Price matching with pharmacy B $140/month (see #13)	(save $120) = $1680
Pharmaceutical coupon $20/month (see #12)	(save $240) = $1440
Transfer prescription 4 times 4 x $20 in store coupons	(save $80) = $1360
Pill splitting (see #14)	(save $680) = $680
Samples from doctor (see #17) 4 x 14 pills = at least 2 months	(save $113) = $567
Final cost: $47/month	$567

Whew!

16. Check out the $4 list

In late 2006 Walmart introduced the "$4 list" of generic prescription medicines. Since then many large retailers have followed suit. For about $4 you can obtain a one-month supply of certain generic drugs. For $10, a three-month supply is available.

Ask your local discount pharmacy if they have such a plan, or go online and do a search for "$4 drugs" or "$3.99 drugs." (See appendix 4 for a list of drugstores with online $4 formularies.)

If you have a prescription plan, your co-pay may be higher than the out-of-pocket cost of the medication. Ask your pharmacist about paying cash if this is the case. Since the pharmacy may actually be paid more through insurance than with these cash prices, you have to speak up.

Hundreds of generic medications are available on these lists, which vary somewhat from pharmacy to pharmacy.

The following is a sampling of medications available on most $4 drug lists:

- Antibiotics (amoxicillin, cephalexin, ciprofloxacin, erythromycin, doxycycline, penicillin, sulfa drugs, tetracycline, and others)
- Antifungals and anti-yeast (fluconazole, terbinafine, several creams)
- Antiviral (acyclovir)
- Arthritis (allopurinol, colchicine, diclofenac, ibupro-

fen, naproxen) (Note: Colchicine may be removed from this list in 2010.)

- Cholesterol (lovastatin, sometimes pravastatin or simvastatin) (Note: Check around, as these vary by pharmacy. If not on your pharmacy's list, ask about price matching.)
- Diabetes (glimepiride, glipizide, glyburide, metformin, and others)
- Eye care (pilocarpine, timolol, eye antibiotic ointments and drops)
- Gastrointestinal (cimetidine, famotidine, ranitidine, promethazine, dicyclomine, metoclopramide, and others)
- Heart and blood pressure (atenolol, benazepril, digoxin, diltiazem, furosemide, lisinopril, nitroglycerin, warfarin, and others)
- Menopause (estrogens and progesterones)
- Mental health (amitriptyline, buspirone, citalopram, doxepin, fluoxetine, lithium, paroxetine, and others)
- Skin care (steroid creams, antifungal creams, burn creams)
- Thyroid (levothyroxine, various strengths)
- Vitamins and minerals (various)

17. Request drug samples

Samples sell. That's the bottom line—at least for pharmaceutical companies.

They want to make money. You, on the other hand, want to save money. Can both these objectives be satisfied?

Even if a drug company never makes a dime from you directly, they benefit indirectly from your doctor's use of samples. If a physician becomes familiar with a medication and has confidence in its results, he or she is more likely to prescribe this same medication for other patients. Voila, the company makes a profit. Just not on you.

Many doctors keep a variety of sample medications on hand, supplied free of cost by the pharmaceutical industry. As a rule, these are brand-name products. These samples are for your use, but odds are, you'll need to ask for them. Your doctor may well be too busy to offer.

So ask. Ask, if you're starting a new medication and want to see if it will work. Ask, if you're concerned about side effects and want to try a medicine for a few days before committing to the purchase. Ask, if on occasion you're waiting for your mail-order prescription. And ask, if you're short on money and have to choose between medicine and your next meal.

Sample amounts range from a single pill to an entire month of therapy (and sometimes a single pill is an entire month of therapy!). Most sample boxes contain four to seven days of medicine. With higher-priced prescriptions this may amount to $20 to $40 of free medicine, often more than the co-pay for your office visit.

Samples of inhalers, patches, and creams are also commonly available. Sample inhalers contain enough medicine for a week to a month of therapy, easily $10 to $50 in savings.

A two-gram sample of a steroid cream may be all you need for a minor rash. Topical pain patches such as the Flector patch are somewhat expensive, but samples are plentiful and a few patches may get you beyond your acute back strain or ankle sprain.

Keep in mind if you start a brand-name medication in the form of samples your doctor is likely to continue the same medication unless you complain about the cost. It may be cheaper in the long run to start (or switch to) an older, generic drug.

18. Look into patient assistance programs

Patient assistance programs are available through the large pharmaceutical companies for low-income, uninsured (or underinsured) Americans. You may qualify for help if your income is less than 200 percent of the Federal Poverty Guidelines. Some programs allow patients with even higher income levels to qualify for free or reduced cost medications.

As of May 2010, the United States Department of Health and Human Services continues to use the 2009 guidelines. In the continental United States, 200 percent of the Federal Poverty Guidelines equals $44,100 for a family of four, $29,140 for a family of two, and $21,660 for an individual. Guidelines for other family sizes, as well as income guidelines for Alaska and Hawaii are listed at: http://aspe.hhs.gov/POVERTY/09poverty .shtml.

Years ago patient assistance programs were available only through your personal physician, but now most are accessible via the Internet. It is not likely your local pharmacy will refer you to a program that is competing for your health care dollar, though some will do so. If your doctor or her staff cannot supply you with the needed information, search online. Presumably you have more time and motivation to do so than does your doctor. Recognizing that doctors do not like to be burdened with additional unpaid work, the pharmaceutical companies have simplified their programs to allow the patient to do the majority of this paperwork.

A quick way to find these programs is through an Internet search for "patient assistance programs" or "prescription assistance programs." Or simply visit the Partnership for Prescription Assistance (PPA) Web site at www.pparx.org. (A Spanish version of the Web site is also available.) As of this writing, the PPA has resources to help patients and providers find discounts for medications from multiple pharmaceutical companies. You may call them at 1-888-4PPA-NOW (1-888-477-2669) Monday through Friday, from 9:00 A.M. to 5:00 P.M. eastern time. This site provides information for help with:

- More than 2,500 medicines
- 475 patient assistance programs

To receive medications under these programs you must first have a written prescription from your doctor. The prescription must be mailed or faxed to the appropriate pharmaceutical company along with documentation of your financial

information. Some companies require you to qualify finan-
cially before they allow you to submit a prescription. You
need to allow at least a few weeks for approval. Once you
qualify for a particular program, you are generally eligible to
receive any medication from that particular pharmaceutical
company at a discounted fee, often at no cost. You may want
to talk to your doctor about whether your prescriptions can
be consolidated to a single drug company's products. Eligibility needs to be redocumented every three to twelve months.
Usually the companies will send a three-month supply of
medication at a time.

The programs do require some effort on your part as well
as that of your physician. Busy doctors may run the other
way if you approach them with a mountain of paperwork. If
you need your doctor to sign a form for you, *please* have your
portion completed and ready to go. If the form needs to be
mailed, *please* have an addressed, stamped envelope prepared ahead of time.

Once you have qualified and submitted your prescription,
the pharmaceutical company will deliver these free or reduced cost products either to you or your designated doctor
via the U.S. postal service, FedEx, or similar carrier. This
may result in packages of medication being left unattended
in your mailbox or on your porch, so watch closely for your
expected delivery.

Having your doctor switch you from a brand-name medication to an appropriate generic may be simpler in the long
run. If she can find an appropriate generic that may be split
as well, your cost may be as low as $20 for an entire year of
medication.

19. Combine pills and save

From jeans to Jaguars, who doesn't like a bargain?

Buy one, get one free. Combination pills work on the same principle—two medications for the price of one, combined into a single pill. You pay for the more expensive of the two, with the second thrown in for free.

Most commonly these products involve two medications from the same therapeutic class, for example, two blood pressure drugs in a single pill. Combination pills are available to treat high blood pressure, diabetes, high cholesterol, and several other common conditions.

This isn't a new idea. Cough and cold preparations have long been concoctions of multiple medications to treat a cluster of symptoms. But in recent years, pharmaceutical companies have produced combination pills, touting the benefits of convenience and lower cost. Originally these combos included a higher-priced brand-name drug combined with an older, inexpensive generic. Nowadays, many exist in generic-generic versions.

You can save a little or save a lot. The "$4 list" includes several options, especially for blood pressure control. Even if you save only $4 a month, that's $48 a year, enough for a night out or a new dress. And saving an extra $20 co-pay each month may amount to over $200 a year.

Research shows patient compliance improves when the number of daily pills is minimized. Most people do well with once-a-day medication and fairly well with twice-a-day. Beyond that, doctors should assume their patients are missing doses.

Let's start with cholesterol medication. Nowadays many people are taking both a statin drug as well as ezetimibe (Zetia). The combination pill, Vytorin, has two ingredients: simvastatin (generic Zocor) and Zetia. The cost of Vytorin is the same as that of Zetia. Buying the combination pill rather than the two separately will save you $48 a year. Plus you only have to remember to take one pill a day.

If you have both high cholesterol and high blood pressure, your doctor may have prescribed atorvastatin (Lipitor) and amlodipine (Norvasc). Caduet contains both these ingredients, at a slightly lower price than the cost of both brand-name drugs combined. For insured patients, this is great: you'll save the cost of one co-pay a month—which could be as much as $50, totaling $600 a year. However, for uninsured patients, your out-of-pocket expense may be lower if you buy the drugs separately: ask your doctor if he's willing to prescribe the Lipitor in a higher-milligram dose so you can split the pill and save 50 percent (see #14).

Many patients are taking more than one blood pressure medication. The $4 list includes beta-blockers combined with diuretics and ACE inhibitors combined with diuretics, another opportunity to save $50 a year.

For diabetes, both pioglitazone (Actos) and rosiglitazone (Avandia) are commonly prescribed with metformin. Actoplus Met is a combination pill that includes Actos plus metformin. Avandamet is Avandia plus metformin. Here again you will save at least $50 a year using the combination drugs. Self-pay patients should compare all doses of these medications online (e.g., at www.drugstore.com) to find which version of the drug will actually be least expensive for you.

Many patients with chronic asthma or COPD are prescribed an inhaled steroid to stabilize their symptoms. Along with this some are prescribed a long-acting bronchodilator. Purchased separately, these two types of drugs would cost well over $200 a month. The combination inhalers Advair and Symbicort offer substantial savings over the separate ingredients. There are no generic equivalents, so all these drugs are expensive. But even insured patients could save $50 a month by avoiding a second co-pay (and don't forget to look online for coupons—see #12). Self-pay patients requiring these medications should check into patient assistance programs (see #18).

Talk to your doctor if you're taking multiple medications for blood pressure, diabetes, cholesterol, allergies, or hormone therapy. He or she may be able to find a suitable cost-saving combination, or perhaps switch you to a similar but equivalent alternative. Combination preparations are also available for certain inhalers, creams, and patches.

The fewer pills the better, I always say. And with the money you save, buy yourself that Jaguar.

20. Kill two birds with one stone: One pill, two effects

If you suffer from multiple problems, a single pill might help more than one condition. This approach may take advantage of the intended benefits of a drug or known side effects.

For example, if you have both *high blood pressure* and *migraine headaches*, a calcium channel blocker may alleviate both conditions.

If you have *hypertension* and *stage fright*, a beta-blocker is the ticket for a calm performance. Beta-blockers not only lower blood pressure, they also slow the heart rate and calm the tremors brought on by too much adrenaline.

Suffering from both rosacea and inflammatory bowel disease? Certain antibiotics may calm both your complexion and your colon. Rosacea is an acne-like eruption of the face that responds to antibiotic therapy. The same antibiotics are sometimes used to lessen the symptoms of colitis as well.

Depressed and hooked on coffin nails? Bupropion may clear the air for you. Years ago an alert observer noticed that some patients taking Wellbutrin (buproprion) for depression were smoking less. Further studies confirmed that the drug is useful in helping smokers quit, leading to the approval of Zyban, the same drug by the same company, repackaged for smoking cessation. If you need an antidepressant and are a smoker, too, ask your doctor about buproprion.

Stressed and got the runs? Appropriate antidepressants may make you smile again. A common side effect of antidepressants is constipation. For the person who tends toward loose stools, this side effect may come in handy.

Overweight and constipated? Orlistat will help you lose more than that extra weight. Prescription or over-the-counter orlistat (Xenical, Alli) is a true fat-blocker, indicated for the treatment of obesity. Most patients experience looser bowels while taking the drug. Although the medicine is not officially indicated for constipation, it will do the job. See #40 for additional information.

Swollen ankles and PMS? Spironolactone may relieve both your physical and mental angst. Spironolactone (Aldactone) is a diuretic (water pill) that provides some quasi-hormonal benefits, such as relief from premenstrual symptoms. It probably would not be your doctor's first choice for relief of swelling, but it is certainly a reasonable choice for a patient with both problems.

Bad back and can't sleep? A muscle relaxer may help you snooze like a baby. Some people can't sleep because their back hurts. Other people just can't sleep. The most common side effect of muscle relaxers is drowsiness. Whereas many patients cannot take these during the day, bedtime use can allow a person to fall asleep more easily, while relieving tight back muscles as well.

High blood pressure and urinate too often? Alpha-blockers may be your ticket to freedom. There are many options for treating high blood pressure. Alpha-blockers are not generally first-line drugs for most hypertensive patients, but they're a great choice for the middle-aged man whose prostate is starting to enlarge, causing urinary frequency, dribbling, or hesitancy. Men, if you're seeing your doctor for high blood pressure and have these urinary symptoms, don't keep it a secret.

Itchy eyes and allergic nose? Antihistamines or nasal inhalers may improve both aggravations. The eyes and the nose are connected via the tear ducts. Cutting down on nasal allergies with a nasal inhaler often helps the eyes as well. Oral antihistamines will help allergy symptoms throughout the body: eyes, nose, skin, and elsewhere.

Heartburn and hives? Ranitidine may calm the acid and eliminate the itch. Certain of the H_2-blockers that are used for decreasing stomach acid also block the histamine effect that results in hives. Though it doesn't work in everyone, it's worth a try for patients with both problems.

Palpitations and hypertension? A beta-blocker or calcium channel blocker may regulate your heart and bring down your blood pressure.

Nauseated and nervous? Vistaril may settle your stomach and brighten your day. Whether you're nauseated from nerves or a stomach bug, hydroxyzine (Vistaril), a mild, non-addicting prescription anxiolytic (anxiety-reliever), can lesson both symptoms.

Ask your doctor whether any of these suggestions would work for you. There are dozens of other ways, perhaps hundreds, to address two problems with one medication. Quite commonly your doctor will suggest such a solution for you.

But if not, don't be afraid to ask. Your doctor may appreciate your inventiveness.

CHAPTER THREE

Save Money on Preventive Health Care

21. A shot in time: Save money on immunizations

In the grand scheme of things, vaccines save money. For society as a whole, immunizing the population generally costs less than treating disease.

The influenza vaccine is a good example of this: the vaccine is inexpensive, is widely available, has few side effects, and is reasonably effective at preventing influenza, especially in susceptible populations at risk for complications and/or hospitalization.

However, certain vaccines can be expensive—nearly $200 for the shingles vaccine. The cost of immunizations continues to be a problem for patients and physicians alike. Some insurance plans reimburse physicians so little that doctors lose money with every vaccine administered. Vaccines cost less when they are purchased in bulk, and insurance often reimburses according to discounted bulk pricing. Yet many doctors cannot buy in bulk, and the vaccines are not returnable for credit. Therefore, many physicians have discontinued giving vaccines until this problem is remedied.

Whereas private doctors pay full price for vaccines, publicly funded clinics and health departments receive special rates. A list of the wholesale cost of vaccines comparing Center for Disease Control (CDC) price versus private sector pricing is available at: www.cdc.gov/vaccines/programs/vfc/cdc-vac-price-list.htm. With government pricing discounts of 30 to 50 percent, it is not possible for the private sector to compete with public clinics and health departments.

The good news? You can take advantage of these government discounts. Don't think of it as welfare—think of it as your tax dollars at work. Check your local health department for details on its immunization clinics. Some of the vaccines are offered to the public free of cost, while others are available at a discounted rate.

However, health departments do not necessarily offer all vaccines, especially not the more expensive ones. In our area they do not offer the chicken pox vaccine, the human papilloma virus vaccine, the shingles vaccine, nor several others.

Here are some additional tips to save money on specific vaccinations.

Tetanus shots: The new "Tdap" costs about $50 whereas the older "Td" is half this amount. The difference has nothing to do with preventing tetanus (lock jaw), but rather pertussis (whooping cough)—which again has nothing to do with an injury. ("T" is for tetanus, "d" is for diphtheria, and "p" is for pertussis.) If you're paying cash (and have good lungs and a good immune system), ask for the older Td.

It was not recognized until recently that adults could get whooping cough. For one thing, they don't usually "whoop." Rather, adults tend to have a prolonged cough, for up to several weeks. In the past it was thought that immunity was lifelong, but now it is understood to lessen within about a decade. Adults ages 19 to 65 who have an underlying breathing problem should probably get the Tdap booster. Another reason for adults to be immunized is to help protect infants in the community from the disease. Otherwise, either vaccine is acceptable, and both are effective at preventing tetanus.

Another way to save money on immunizations is by keeping your tetanus shots up-to-date. Any time you see a doctor is an opportunity to update your tetanus shot. If you wait until you're injured, your doctor will likely want to see you, even if the injury is minor. Why? As mentioned above, doctors often lose money on vaccines. Charging an office call is the only way to make a profit (or perhaps break even) on immunization.

HPV vaccine: Human papilloma virus is sexually transmitted—you cannot contract HPV from a virgin. The series of three shots costs about $360 . . . likely not enough to inspire celibacy. And, of course, the vaccine protects against only certain strains of human papilloma virus—and *does not* protect against AIDS, gonorrhea, syphilis, or any other STD. The vaccine is most effective before the first sexual encounter. Some insurance will cover this vaccine; others won't.

For young women who are celibate, who intend to remain that way, and who plan to marry another like-minded individual, the vaccine should not be necessary. If both partners are virgins, the risk of HPV is essentially nil. (But can you be sure?)

For women who are sexually active, especially those who have more than one sexual partner over time, spending the $360 may save the cost of repeat Pap smears (when an abnormality is detected), a colposcopy ($500 to $1,000), possible HPV treatment, not to mention worrying about the possibility of HPV leading to cervical cancer.

Shingles: As mentioned, the cost of the shingles vaccine is nearly $200. But treating shingles can cost significantly more: the time and expense of one or more office visits, plus medication that can run over $200, plus the potential for chronic pain. In retrospect, the majority of my patients who've had shingles (varicella zoster) wish they'd had the vaccine. Because the incidence of shingles increases with age, this vaccine is indicated for people age 60 and older, and may be covered under Medicare Part D.

The cost-effectiveness of the shingles vaccine is still being debated. Many individuals feel $200 is a small price to pay to prevent what is often a painful disease. But what's the likelihood of coming down with shingles, anyway? For adults under the age of 50, the incidence is about 2 in 1,000 per year. By age 80 that number rises to at least 1 in 100 annually. Doctors need to immunize about 60 patients to prevent one case of shingles over the subsequent three years, yielding a cost of $12,000 to society to prevent one case of shingles. Decide for yourself whether these numbers convince you to get the vaccine.

Keep your own records: If you're at risk of a vaccine-preventable disease and can't provide documentation of vaccination, you'll need blood testing to determine your immune status, or you'll receive a potentially duplicate vaccine—or both. This occurs most commonly when employers require proof of immunization against tetanus, hepatitis, measles, mumps, rubella, and chicken pox. Keep your own record of all your immunizations from birth onward, *forever*. Not only is this information useful for your doctor, it may help you avoid the expense of additional testing or unneeded vaccines.

22. Plan for Paps

Who, when, why? Not everybody. Not every year. Not anymore.

The Pap smear is a screening test for cancer of the cervix—not for sexually transmitted diseases (STDs), other than human papilloma virus (HPV). HPV causes changes in the cells of the cervix (dysplasia or intraepithelial abnormalities). These changes sometimes progress to cervical cancer. The goal of a Pap smear is to detect abnormalities at an early state, when treatment is most effective and least involved— and least expensive.

Who contracts cervical cancer? Although women in their forties and fifties are most at risk for full-blown cancer, the disease is thought to begin much earlier. Younger women often contract the human papilloma virus, which then causes progressive changes in the cervix and may eventually culminate in cancer. For this reason and because early cellular changes can be detected and treated, younger women should receive regular Pap smears.

There is good news, however: in the past Pap smears were

recommended *annually* for every woman. Now *less frequent* testing is recommended, according to a better understanding of the disease process.

Current Recommendations for Pap Smears

- Begin Pap smears within the first three years after a woman's first vaginal intercourse, or age 21, whichever comes first (but see below);
- Continue yearly thereafter using the regular Pap smear, or every two or three years using the ThinPrep Pap, until age 30;
- After age 30, screen women every three years in patients who have had three normal Pap smears in a row, unless the patient is high risk (see www.cancer.org).

The above guidelines, found at www.ahrq.gov/clinic/3rd uspstf/cervcan/cervcanrr.htm, are based on typical American behavior. According to the U.S. Preventive Services Task Force (USPSTF), "Although there is little value in screening women who have never been sexually active, many U.S. organizations recommend routine screening by age 18 or 21 for all women, based on the generally high prevalence of sexual activity by that age in the United States and concerns that clinicians may not always obtain accurate sexual histories." Therefore, it is possible to save money on Pap smears by being 100 percent abstinent.

Because Pap smears sometimes give false-positive or false-negative results, doctors have looked for a better screening test. For this reason a new type of Pap smear was developed several years ago, the liquid-based cervical cytology test, such as the ThinPrep Pap. However, a large study published in the *Journal of the American Medical Association* in 2009 did not confirm that the liquid-based cervical cytology test yielded superior results. The U.S. Preventive Services Task Force currently concludes that there is insufficient evidence to recommend for or against these new Pap smears. Nor do they recommend for or against the use of HPV testing as a primary screening test for cervical cancer.

Next, when should a woman stop getting Pap smears? Again, based on a better understanding of the disease, the USPSTF advises that women may stop Pap smears at:

- Age 65 or 70, in a patient with three prior normal Paps within the last 10 years, unless the patient is at high risk; or
- After a complete hysterectomy, unless the hysterectomy was done for cancer

Putting this all together, you can save money on Pap smears by:

- Not having sex
- Not having a Pap smear more often than needed
- Not having the more costly ThinPrep Pap
- Not having HPV testing unless you are at high risk
- Going to a publicly funded clinic
- Checking out the National Breast and Cervical Cancer

Early Detection Program for uninsured women at: http://apps.nccd.cdc.gov/cancercontacts/nbccedp/contactlist.asp

Know which Pap smear is right for you. Ask your doctor ahead of time which test she plans to do and why. If you're monogamous and healthy, and have had normal Paps in the past, the standard test is appropriate and costs the least.

> The standard Pap smear costs about $55.*
>   The newer ThinPrep costs about $85.*
>   HPV testing runs an additional $170 or more.*
>   *In addition to your doctor's exam fee, another $50 to $150.

23. Minimize your mammogram expense

As of November 2009, mammograms to screen for breast cancer are now recommended every *two years* for all women *ages 50 to 74*, according to the U.S. Preventive Services Task Force (USPSTF). Before that, *annual* testing from *age 40 upward* was recommended.

The USPSTF took a lot of heat for revising the recommendation. Why the change? Low-risk women in their forties are much less likely to have breast cancer than women aged fifty and older. Moreover, mammograms in this younger age group are more likely to yield a false-positive test result, one that could lead to unnecessary X-rays and biopsies, not to mention unnecessary worry.

Does this mean that women in their forties cannot or should not receive a mammogram? No. The USPSTF recommendations encourage women in their forties to talk with their doctors about what is best for them personally. A woman with a strong family history of breast cancer would be encouraged to get a mammogram at a younger age than a person without a similar history.

The current recommendations regarding screening mammograms may be found online at: www.ahrq.gov/clinic/uspstf/uspsbrca.htm.

What is a mammogram, anyway, and why get one at all? A mammogram is a special, low-dose X-ray that shows the detailed structure of soft tissues (as opposed to bones). Cancer appears different from regular fat or glandular tissue, although the mammographic shadow-pictures are not 100 percent precise. Sometimes normal tissue may look abnormal, or vice versa. The intent of a mammogram is to detect small cancers that can be treated more easily than large cancers. A small cancer may only require removing the tumor (a lumpectomy). A larger cancer may require removal of the breast (a mastectomy), radiation, and/or chemotherapy . . . all *very* expensive.

For low-risk patients, getting fewer mammograms is certainly a cost savings, on the order of $80 to $150 per test.

But even women in their forties who opt for annual mammograms can still save money. Few people are aware that free mammograms are available in every state. If you are age 40 to 64, are uninsured or underinsured, and earn less than

200–250 percent of the poverty level (which totals about $27,000 for an individual), you should qualify. The National Breast and Cervical Cancer Early Detection Program offers free breast cancer screening for uninsured and underinsured women *ages 40 to 64*, despite the above change in screening recommendations. Check their Web site for your own state at: http://apps.nccd.cdc.gov/cancercontacts/nbccedp/contact list.asp.

For women age 65 and above, Medicare covers mammograms, subject to a 20 percent co-pay of the approved amount with no Part B deductible. The USPSTF concludes that the current evidence is "insufficient to assess the additional benefits and harms of screening mammography in women 75 years or older." However, Medicare still covers mammograms for this age group.

Additional ways to find free or reduced mammograms include checking with your city or county health department. Or call your local hospital or medical school. Or do an Internet search for "free mammograms in *YourArea*."

Also, keep your eye open for health fairs, especially during the month of October, Breast Cancer Awareness Month. During this month many communities offer mammograms free or at reduced cost. To find a program in your area, call the Susan G. Komen for the Cure Breast Care Helpline at 1-800 I'M AWARE (1-800-462-9273) or visit www.komen.org.

So go get your mammogram. Now there's no excuse.

24. Skip the annual physical?

Just what is an annual physical, anyway?

From a doctor's point of view, the annual physical is an opportunity to detect *but not necessarily discuss or treat* problems and to address issues of "health maintenance," such as exercise, diet, and immunizations—things to keep you healthy. It may also include "routine" labs, X-rays, or an electrocardiogram (EKG).

From a patient's point of view, the visit is often seen as an opportunity to detect, *discuss and treat* everything that may be wrong.

The difference is reflected in different medical billing codes. The billing code for a physical exam reflects only the time spent taking a history and performing the physical. It does not include payment for time spent addressing problems. To be paid to treat problems, a doctor must submit additional "evaluation and management" codes. Also, explaining and treating problems requires additional time, time that may not have been scheduled.

The problem is further complicated by insurance plans. Some pay for annual physicals, some don't. Some pay for treating problems at the same visit, some won't. The physical may count against your deductible, or not. *Very confusing.* With the passage of the 2010 Health Reform Bill, there will be more changes forthcoming regarding payment for preventive care visits.

So before you schedule a physical, ask yourself why you're going. What benefit do you hope to derive and what's it worth to you? A "complete physical" could easily run $150 or more.

From a medical standpoint, in a healthy individual there's nothing sacred about a yearly physical—ask your doctor whether the same benefit could be gained from exams every two, three, even five years.

For women who undergo periodic exams for Pap smears or birth control, ask your doctor if a separate physical is advisable. As a family doctor, I do a fairly complete exam at the time of a Pap and use this opportunity to address other issues. (Gynecologists, on the other hand, will likely focus on only issues within their domain of female health.)

If the real reason you want to see your doctor is because you have a problem—or several—don't schedule a physical, make an appointment to address your problems instead. Read #1, 2, 3, 5, 6, 9, 55, and 57 for more ideas on saving money on exams.

The value you hope to gain from seeing a doctor should be clear to both you and your physician. Ideally this is discussed when you schedule your appointment or within the first few minutes of your visit. Your doctor wants to help you—and it helps your doctor do so when she knows why you've come and what you're looking for.

25. Sports and work physicals

Most people just want a rubber stamp of approval when they come to the doctor for a physical for work or to play sports. But if you're on a budget, perhaps you'd like more value for your health care dollar.

For those of you with insurance, sports and work physicals will not be covered under your plan but an annual physical may be. Check the particulars before you call to schedule. Your doctor may be willing to fill out your sports or work physical form as part of a covered exam.

Think ahead. If your teenager needs a sports physical now but will need a work physical later (or vice versa), consider combining the two. At least in Ohio the sports physical examination is more comprehensive than a work-permit exam—the work-permit form could easily be completed at the time of a sports physical, but the opposite is not true. If your teen undergoes a brief work-permit exam, he or she will have to return for the longer sports physical. Since the exams are generally valid for a year, plan ahead.

You get what you pay for. A thorough sports physical from your private pediatrician could be an opportunity to update immunizations, discuss issues regarding puberty, drug or alcohol use, or other concerns. If your child has a chronic health condition such as asthma, your personal physician will do what she can to make it safe for your child to participate in sports.

Sports physicals are often available for under $50, provided as a community service through your local hospital, a physician's office, a clinic, a health department, or an urgent care center. Sometimes a doctor or group of doctors will perform physicals at your child's school. These exams are quick, cheap, and probably appropriate for the healthy kid who's already been playing for years. But if any problem is found, your child will be referred back to your personal physician for clearance and treatment, costing you more in the long run.

Some work physicals are paid for by the employer. In this situation he who pays dictates what's done, but you or your doctor may be able to get a copy of any tests and blood work that are included. Ask whether you're entitled to a copy of your physical as well—it's possible your employer-paid work physical could be substituted for an annual physical from your doctor.

If you're hoping to add a sports or work physical to a visit for an acute problem, *please* call and ask first (see #5). Your doctor might be willing but may well refuse unless you make arrangements ahead of time.

26. Colon cancer screening: To scope or not to scope?

You're over 50. You don't want colon cancer. And you don't have the $1,500 to $2,000 for a screening colonoscopy. What's a person to do?

If you're between 50 and 75 years old, colon cancer screening is recommended (or younger if you have a family history of colon cancer or polyps). For adults between the ages of 76 and 85, the U.S. Preventive Services Task Force recommends *against* screening for colon cancer, except in individual patients with special considerations. At age 86 and above, *no colon cancer screening* is recommended. The guidelines are available online at: www.ahrq.gov/clinic/usp stf/uspscolo.htm.

In recent years there's been a trend for doctors to recommend colonoscopy (every ten years) as the test of choice to detect early colon cancer. No doubt fear of missing something (and resultant malpractice litigation) is part of the reason.

But though colonoscopy does have the greatest accuracy for a single test, it's not the only option. The flexible sigmoidoscopy (a similar test with a shorter scope) performed every five years is nearly as effective at finding colon cancer early enough to extend one's life. A flexible sigmoidoscopy costs about $400 (a total of $800 per decade), a savings of $700 to $1,600 versus colonoscopy.

But cheaper yet is annual fecal occult blood analysis, which tests for microscopic levels of blood in the stool. Colon cancer often bleeds, even early on, and can be detected before other symptoms occur. At about $30 a year, or $300 a decade, this is a proven and cost-effective alternative to colonoscopy. However, if blood is detected, you'll still need to have a colonoscopy.

One thing you don't want to do is have a false-positive test that may necessitate the more expensive colonoscopy. A fecal occult blood test is sensitive enough to detect blood from red meat eaten as much as two days beforehand. And aspirin and other NSAIDs (see #96) sometimes cause the stomach to bleed—so avoiding such NSAIDs and red meat for two days before testing is also recommended.

Another concern is hemorrhoids. If you have hemorrhoids and know they're bleeding, that would not be a good time to do fecal occult blood testing. The test will be positive and your doctor will want you to have a colonoscopy. Heal your hemorrhoids (see #89) and wait a week or two before obtaining the needed stool samples.

Insurance and Medicare may pay for colon cancer screening, but it would be wise to check your benefit coverage before scheduling any test. For more information visit www .familydoctor.org and do a search for "colon cancer."

27. Prostate cancer screening: Can you buy peace of mind with a PSA?

My friend has prostate cancer. Shouldn't I be tested, too? That depends.

According to the U.S. Preventive Services Task Force (USPSTF), there isn't enough evidence to conclude whether the benefit outweighs the harm, at least in men younger than 75. For men 75 years or older the USPSTF recommends *against* screening for prostate cancer.

How is that possible? The problem with prostate cancer is lots of men get it (up to 25 percent) but few men die from it (only 3 percent). And at least in older men, treatment doesn't usually prolong a person's life.

It's true the PSA (Prostate Specific Antigen) test can detect early cancer, before a man experiences any symptoms. Unfortunately, the test also carries a risk of false-positive results. It may look like you have prostate cancer when in reality you don't. In fact, for every four men who have an elevated PSA suggestive of prostate cancer, only one will have the disease, according to the Mayo Clinic. But you won't know the result is a false-positive without a biopsy and further testing. That's more money.

The USPSTF Web site at www.ahrq.gov/clinic/uspstf/uspsprca.htm features a video (intended for doctors) that may help you understand these recommendations better (*How to Talk with Your Patients When Evidence Is Insufficient*). For a detailed explanation of the pros and cons of PSA testing, visit the Mayo Clinic Web site at www.mayoclinic .com/health/prostate-cancer/HQ01273.

If treatment for prostate cancer were simple, effective, and free of side effects, then everyone should be treated. Unfortunately, impotence and urinary leakage are common side effects of treatment, enough to make a man think twice.

Will a $90 PSA test buy you peace of mind? Not if you're one with a false-positive result. So if you'd rather not spend your hard-earned money on a PSA test, it's OK. If your doctor says you should do so, ask him why, exactly. But if your father, brother, or son has had prostate cancer, you should be tested. Otherwise, it's your preference, whether to do it at all, every year, or every now and then.

Also, if you have insurance but no symptoms to suggest prostate cancer, check your coverage ahead of time—a PSA test may not be covered.

Checking for prostate cancer in a person *with* symptoms is another matter altogether. See your doctor if any of the following occur:

- A change in the urine stream
- Difficulty starting to urinate

- Dribbling after urination
- Frequent urination
- Blood or pus in the urine or semen
- Pain while urinating or ejaculating
- Persistent low-back or pelvic pain
- Weight loss or loss of appetite

28. Cholesterol screening: Free and low-cost testing

I'm afraid my cholesterol is high but I can't afford to pay for blood tests.

At a cost of about $100, a fasting lipid profile from a medical lab provides the most complete picture. This profile generally includes total cholesterol, HDL and LDL cholesterol, and triglycerides. That's about the same cost as a year of oil changes. Is your car worth more than your health?

Individual tests for total or LDL cholesterol run under $50, and "quick" tests cost considerably less (also somewhat less accurate, but still useful).

Free or discounted cholesterol screens are frequently offered at health fairs, health departments, pharmacies, and

Winn-Dixie offers free cholesterol and diabetes testing at their pharmacies. For more information, check their Web site at: www.winndixie.com/Health/Health_Wellness.asp.

Walgreens and AARP have joined together in

2009–2010 to offer free testing to communities across the country. The free screenings include: total cholesterol level, blood pressure, bone density, glucose level, waist circumference, and body mass index. Check the schedule for your state at: www.walgreens.com/topic/health-screenings/bus-tour.jsp or call 1-866-484-8687.

hospitals (see #55 and #57). Blood and plasma donation sites often offer a free cholesterol test as an incentive to donate.

Home cholesterol testing is available and inexpensive. The *ADA CheckUP America American Diabetes Association Cholesterol Panel* (sold for under $50) allows you to mail a blood sample for a complete lipid panel without a doctor's order. Patients obtain the sample at home by pricking their finger, then mail the sample to an approved lab. Test results are available at a secure Web site or by mail. Pharmacies also sell simpler in-home tests for total cholesterol costing under $20.

Remember, high cholesterol is not a *disease* in itself. It's a *risk factor* for heart disease and stroke. You can lower your risk without even knowing your cholesterol. First off, quit smoking. (Just think of all the money you'll save!) It makes little sense to worry about your cholesterol if you won't quit smoking. Secondly, eat a low-fat diet. I've had patients lower their cholesterol 50 points or more with diet alone. Third, get regular aerobic exercise, at least 30 minutes of walking three–five times a week. And fourth, lose weight. Even 15–20 pounds can make a difference. Lastly, if you're a male and over age 50, take an aspirin a day.

29. Osteoporosis screening: Balancing your bones and your budget

Medicare and most insurance pay for bone-density testing every two years in women with a valid diagnosis code. But for those of you paying your own way, you're probably concerned about the $200 to $400 a DEXA scan would cost.

My rule of thumb is, get the test if it will make a difference in treatment, but don't if it won't.

First you need to understand this: bones are not static, like a piece of plastic. From birth onward, bones undergo constant remodeling. Calcium goes in and calcium comes out. Early on, the gain outweighs the loss. Later, the loss outweighs the gain—especially after menopause.

There are two aspects to keeping bones strong: ensuring a good calcium supply and preventing excess loss.

All women need about 1,500 milligrams of dietary calcium (along with vitamin D) from food or supplements. (No, a once daily vitamin does not contain enough calcium.) Everybody, even those taking additional medicine, needs to replenish his or her calcium daily. A DEXA scan does not tell you whether you need calcium—you do, period. *Everybody does.*

Secondly, certain medications help prevent the loss of calcium. These include hormones, bisphosphonates, and others, at a cost of $4 to over $100 a month. A DEXA test may actually *save* you money if you find you don't need medicine.

On the other hand, if you're at risk for osteoporosis anyway, you should probably be taking one of these medicines, regardless of testing. Ask your doctor if a scan would change his or her recommendation one way or the other.

As of 2010 the question as to how long to take a bisphosphonate for treatment or prevention of osteoporosis is under debate. Fosamax, Boniva, Actonel, and equivalent generics slow the turnover of calcium in bones, and as a result, keep more calcium in the bones. However, the micro-architecture of the bones turns out to appear older and therefore the bones may be more fragile. Taking these medicines longer than five years may be counterproductive, but additional research is required. Whether intermittent use would be advisable also requires further study. Ask your doctor for the latest information.

Physician-ordered DEXA scans check the bones at risk for significant and debilitating fracture: the spine and hip. Less expensive testing at health fairs generally scans the heel, wrist, or finger. A normal result may be reassuring, but an abnormal test indicates the need for a full scan (or treatment).

The U.S. Preventive Services Task Force recommends routine screening for all women aged 65 and older. Women at increased risk for weak bones should begin screening at age 60. There are no specific guidelines for women younger than age 60, although I would recommend patients on certain medications such as corticosteroids be screened much earlier—also patients with a strong family history of osteoporosis, or someone who has suffered a fracture with only minimal trauma. There are no USPSTF recommendations regarding men, since they are much less at risk of osteoporosis due to their heavier bone mass.

If you're under 65 and taking calcium (with vitamin D) and hormones (for whatever reason), there's no rush to get a scan—you're already on an acceptable treatment regimen for prevention of osteoporosis.

Weight-bearing exercise, such as walking, is also known to keep weight-bearing bones (back and leg bones) stronger. A minimum of twenty minutes a day is reasonable for bone and cardiovascular health. People with advanced osteoporosis, however, should be very cautious, as collapse of bones in the spine (vertebral compression fractures) can occur with minimal exertion. Ask your doctor for specific recommendations at your next checkup.

30. Carotid artery screening: When it makes sense and when it doesn't

Not having a problem? Skip the test.

Direct-to-consumer marketing lures many middle-aged and senior adults to pay out of pocket for tests their doctors have not ordered. But are these tests worth your hard-earned money? Not likely.

Carotid artery ultrasonography is only a *screening* test. By definition a screening test is an examination performed on a population of people not known to have the problem in question. Some might call it looking for trouble, but screening tests *are* valuable when the expected good outweighs the potential harm. Unfortunately, when many people are tested, there's always some harm.

No test is perfect, and ultrasound testing of the arteries in the neck is a long way from it. Though the test can detect stenosis (narrowing or obstruction) of the arteries, ultrasonography cannot predict who will and who won't have a stroke.

A negative test might be reassuring, but its accuracy cannot be guaranteed.

A positive test may lead your doctor to order angiography (with its 1 percent risk of stroke) or even refer you for surgery (with a higher risk of stroke).

But we're trying to prevent strokes, right?

Risk factors for carotid artery stenosis (and stroke) include high blood pressure, high cholesterol, heart disease, tobacco use, older age, and male sex. Though in a person with multiple risk factors screening might be more useful, the same risk factors that predispose to carotid artery stenosis are also risk factors for surgical complications.

The U.S. Preventive Services Task Force has concluded that for persons without symptoms, there's no proof the benefits of screening outweigh the harm. So if you are symptom free, skip the test.

Now, if you *are* having intermittent symptoms suggesting a stroke or mini-stroke, you need to *see your doctor*, who will order several tests in addition to an ultrasound of your carotid arteries (tests that Medicare and insurance will pay for).

Symptoms suggestive of a stroke include sudden weakness in an arm or a leg, or both (usually on the same side), drooping or numbness of one side of the face, difficulty talking, sudden change in memory or vision, sudden severe headache, or dizziness or falling. You should go to the emergency room or call 911 if you experience sudden onset of these symptoms. If the symptoms occur but then subside, you still may have suffered a mini-stroke and should call your doctor immediately. Patients who have mild symptoms that come and go are also at risk and should consult their doctor. A community-based screening is not a sufficient evaluation.

But if you're not having symptoms, *be thankful!* Don't smoke, lower your cholesterol and blood pressure (see #38–#40), take an aspirin if your doctor suggests it, and stop worrying.

CHAPTER FOUR

Save Money on Chronic Health Problems

31. Allergies: Don't sneeze at these savings

Get rid of the cat and maybe you won't need medication. Seriously. Or the dog, or the bird.

Stay away from dust, mold, plants, trees, animals, food, and air and you should be allergy-free. You won't need medicine and you won't need a doctor.

If you can't avoid your triggers completely, at least keep pets out of your bedroom, shower after mowing the grass, rinse out your nose with a netty pot, and keep your house free of dust and mold.

But if you do need medicine, save money by knowing the right drug to help your symptoms.

Antihistamines decrease secretions, drying up a drippy nose or postnasal drainage, which often causes cough. They also decrease itching of the eyes, nose, and skin. Several cost only $4 to $10. (See #97 for a longer discussion of antihistamines.) Traditionally antihistamines have been taken orally (by mouth), but now antihistamine nose sprays and eye drops are available to treat localized symptoms.

If you read the fine print regarding over-the-counter and prescription antihistamine usage, you may find a warning against using these if you have asthma. For patients with *allergic* asthma, this is not necessarily true—consult your doctor for additional information.

Decongestants open the airways by reducing swelling in the tissues lining the nose, sinuses, and bronchial tubes. Pseudoephedrine (the original Sudafed) is among the most effective and is the active ingredient in prescription decongestants. It is also available over the counter, but you'll have to ask the pharmacist for it. Generic is effective and costs only $4–$10. Some insurance will actually cover the OTC drug if your doctor writes a prescription for it. Patients with high blood pressure, heart disease, or palpitations should consult their doctor before using decongestants, which sometimes worsen these conditions.

When your nose is totally stuffed up, use Afrin or similar generic for quick relief—but only for a day or two. Longer use tends to cause the nose to become dependent on the medication, a problem that may require prescription medication to overcome.

Nasal steroids (Flonase, Veramyst, Rhinocort, Nasonex, fluticasone) and cromolyn sodium (NasalCrom) all help prevent nasal congestion, itching, and drainage by making the nose less reactive to allergic stimulants (allergens). Only NasalCrom is available over the counter and also costs much less: only $15–$20 versus over $100 for brand-name prescription nasal steroids.

One advantage of using the nasal preparations is avoiding the side effects of antihistamines and decongestants. In general, antihistamines tend to cause drowsiness whereas decongestants have caffeine-like effects (insomnia, rapid heart rate). Interestingly, some people get the opposite reaction.

Expectorants (primarily guaifenesin) thin mucus, making it easier for secretions to drain or to be coughed out (expectorated). Guaifenesin is the active ingredient in Mucinex, as well as many cough and sinus preparations. Expectorants are commonly used in conjunction with decongestants or cough suppressants.

Cough suppressants (primarily dextromethorphan) decrease the brain's sensitivity to the stimulus to cough. Sometimes this is the right approach, but coughs that are due to drainage may benefit from antihistamines, decongestants, nose sprays, or expectorants. Some allergic coughs are related to asthma and benefit from asthma medications (see #33).

OTC (over-the-counter) drugs are excellent and most were by prescription in recent years. Check these Web sites for current offers on prescription and over-the-counter medications.

www.afrin.com

www.allegra.com

www.benadryl.com

www.clarinex.com

www.claritin.com

www.mucinex.com

www.nasacort.com

www.nasonex.com

www.palgic.com

www.pataday.com

www.robitussin.com

www.singulair.com

www.sudafed.com

www.veramyst.com

www.xyzal.com

www.zyrtec.com

32. Arthritis: Soothe your aching bones

By far the most common type of arthritis is osteoarthritis, also called *degenerative* arthritis, or regular old arthritis that everybody gets with aging. For patients with *inflammatory* arthritis such as rheumatoid or lupus, initial treatment for mild cases is often the same as for degenerative arthritis.

You can save money using either prescription or OTC drugs, but since these medications can have serious side effects, talk to your doctor before using them. For many patients Tylenol works as well as anything, is safe at recommended doses, and has fewer side effects.

Over-the-counter or prescription anti-inflammatory drugs (NSAIDs) not only help relieve the pain of arthritis, they can reduce swelling and inflammation as well. All NSAIDs have the potential to irritate the stomach or cause ulcers, although celecoxib (Celebrex) is less likely to do so. In general, the less of these medicines, the better. But they do help, often better than anything else. (See #96 for a lengthier discussion of NSAID medications.)

For people who cannot tolerate anti-inflammatory drugs by mouth, there are now two topical NSAID preparations, Voltaren Gel and the Flector Patch, both of which are more expensive than generic pills. These are most appropriate for patients with limited areas of arthritis rather than a large number of inflamed joints. Check for coupons at their respective Web sites, www.voltarengel.com and www.flector.com.

Many patients do well with medication that only relieves pain (as opposed to relieving inflammation). Beyond Tylenol, tramadol is an effective choice and is not addictive. The short-acting, immediate-release version is on the $4 list. Brand-name tramadol is also available in a long-acting form, Ultram-ER, which has recently gone generic as well. As of early 2010, a month's supply of the 200-milligram once-a-day name-brand medication costs over $200, with the generic running about $130. Personally, for a savings of over $120, I'd opt for taking the short-acting pill more frequently.

Most patients do not require stronger (narcotic) medication. The long-acting forms are quite expensive and best avoided. You don't want to add addiction to your arthritis.

Sometimes, for an individual with one or two inflamed joints, doctors recommend that the patient undergo steroid joint injections. Injections are quite effective at relieving local symptoms, and avoid the problems associated with long-term systemic corticosteroids (weight gain, weakened bones, appetite changes, elevated blood sugar). A single joint injection costs about $50 to $100, depending on the joint. Large joints may cost more. *Occasionally*, short-term treatment with oral steroids is an alternative, at a cost of under $10.

Rheumatoid arthritis sometimes requires treatment beyond any of the above. If your insurance is paying, you may not object to a prescription for Humira, costing $1,700 per box. If your doctor believes this is absolutely the best medication for you, visit www.humira.com for ways for insured, uninsured, and Medicare patients to save. Likewise, you may balk at paying $800 to $1,700 for a month of Enbrel, but the manufacturer also offers help with payment at www.enbrel.com. Another of the expensive arthritic medications is Arava, at a cost of over $600 month. Fortunately, it is now available in generic, but a word of caution: check around—the price for generic may vary from $64 a month to over $400! Hopefully, doctors are ordering these medications only when the benefit clearly outweighs the cost.

Recent advertisements may lead you to believe that Humira and Enbrel are the only options for rheumatoid arthritis. Hydroxychloroquine sulfate (Plaquenil) and methotrexate (Rheumatrex) are older medications that are both available in generic form for under $40 a month.

Gout is another common form of arthritis that responds to NSAID medication. Usually gout affects the feet, with exquisite tenderness of the big toe. Although allopurinol (Zyloprim) has been on the market for decades, many people are still unaware that medication exists *to prevent* this painful condition. Generic allopurinol sells for $30 to $60 a month. A year of preventive medicine is cheaper than a single trip to the emergency room.

Colchicine is also used to treat acute gout. As of early 2010, it is available in generic for about $25 for 30 pills, whereas brand-name colchicine (Colcrys) runs about $165. However, the generic is expected to be unavailable later this year, so if you need this medication, ask your doctor about stocking up now. Another option is to check into the Colcrys Patient Assistance Program, which offers significant discounts for patients with an annual household income up to six times the Federal Poverty Level. (Visit www .colcrys.com.)

Medication is not the only therapy for arthritis. Other low-cost interventions include:

- Appropriate rest
- Exercise, especially stretching and swimming
- Weight loss and a healthy diet
- Supports and braces for painful knees, ankles, and wrists
- Heat and/or ice, 20–30 minutes, two–four times daily
- Good shoes
- A good laugh

33. Asthma and COPD: Spend less and breathe easier

The goal of asthma therapy is *normal* lung function. Patients with chronic asthma often become content with *subnormal* lung function, forgetting what it is to breathe normally.

The goal of chronic obstructive lung disease (COPD) therapy is *optimized* lung function and prevention of flares (exacerbations). Permanent damage may already have occurred and normal lung function may not be achievable for patients with COPD. However, *every* COPD patient has the potential for some improvement. Help yourself achieve these goals by:

- Not smoking
- Avoiding second-hand smoke and other pollutants
- Avoiding allergy triggers (pollen, dust, mold, pets, etc.)
- Getting an annual flu shot
- Getting a pneumonia vaccine if advised by your physician
- Avoiding people with colds and other respiratory infections
- Exercising regularly
- Taking your medication as prescribed
- Knowing your personal peak flow rates (have your doctor review this with you)

Don't skimp on medications. Many asthmatic patients do not have their disease well controlled because they do not take their medications properly. Reasons for this include cost concerns, inadequate understanding of the disease, and the belief that their symptoms are insufficient to warrant treatment.

Talk to your doctor to determine the best regimen for you personally. If finances are a concern, work with your doctor to find medication you can afford. The patient assistance programs (see #18) can help you obtain free medication in certain instances.

Albuterol is prescribed for nearly every asthmatic and COPD patient, intended for occasional or as-needed use. Doctors often refer to albuterol as a "rescue inhaler," meaning it should only be used when symptoms are insufficiently relieved by a "controller medication." Many patients overuse albuterol because it is less expensive than controller medicines and because it works so quickly.

Albuterol HFA (the handheld metered-dose inhaler) is available as Ventolin, Proventil, and ProAir (a branded generic). These inhalers sell for $45 to $55. Interestingly, some pharmacies actually sell the brand-name products for less than the branded generic. Of these three, Ventolin is the only device that includes a counter, so that you'll know how much medication remains in the canister, a very useful feature. In order to get the best deal on albuterol, you need to know your formulary (see #11) if you have insurance, and you need to check with your pharmacy regarding their pricing structure.

Don't forget to ask your doctor for samples or coupons, or check for special offers online (at www.proventilhfa.com, www.ventolin.com, or www.proairhfa.com). Even insured patients can save hundreds of dollars a year on co-pays. Pharmacists may have coupons on hand as well.

If you're paying full price for your albuterol, ask your doctor about Ventolin ReliOn, a $9, 60-dose brand-name albuterol inhaler available at only Walmart and Target. True, it will take three of these to equal one standard albuterol inhaler, but still that's only $27, half the price of a full-sized inhaler. Doctors can write a prescription for the pharmacy to dispense three inhalers at a time, requiring a single co-pay for insured patients.

If that's still too costly, talk to your doctor about using a nebulizer instead. Why would you spend $50 to $100 for a breathing machine when you want to save money? Because the medication used in a nebulizer is so inexpensive. Both albuterol and ipratropium nebulizer solutions are on the $4 list, much cheaper than handheld metered-dose inhalers. Your doctor may not be aware of this, so be sure to bring it up. Substituting home nebulizer treatments for *some* doses of an inhaler may save you hundreds of dollars annually. You'll still want to keep a rescue inhaler handy, however, for when you're away from your machine. Nebulizers are available at your pharmacy or online (www.drugstore.com and elsewhere), and are commonly covered by insurance (see #72).

Asthma medications on the $4 list include:

- Albuterol tablets, syrup, and nebulizer solution in bottles and single dose vials
- Dexamethasone tablets

- Ipratropium 0.02 percent nebulizer solution in single dose vials
- Prednisone pills and dose paks
- Ventolin ReliOn albuterol inhaler ($9 for 60-dose inhaler, sold at only Walmart and Target)

The Maxair Autohaler (pirbuterol) is another rescue inhaler packaged in an easy to use device. At this time it does not have a generic form and runs over $100 for a single inhaler. However, for patients who have difficulty coordinating their breathing with the administration of a traditional albuterol inhaler, it's a great option.

Some patients may be tempted to use an over-the-counter asthma inhaler. Please don't unless your doctor specifically advises you to do so—*which he won't.* They can be dangerous.

The next class of drugs is the controller medications, intended to stabilize asthma. These include inhaled steroids, long-acting beta-agonists, leukotriene inhibitors, and theophylline. This is another instance where knowing your formulary may save you money on Advair, Symbicort, Spiriva, Singulair, Flovent, Azmacort, Pulmicort, and Serevent. Each of these medicines is expensive, but help is available. Self-pay patients should check online for coupons and patient assistance programs, as described in #18.

Another option is the older medication theophylline. Before inhaled steroids, before Singulair, before ipratropium, there was theophylline, the mainstay of asthma therapy. This medication is still available, is quite inexpensive, and is effective for many patients. There are drawbacks—drug interactions, the need for periodic blood monitoring, jitteriness, nausea in some patients, and concerns with overdose—*but* for patients on a budget it is a consideration, and can save $1,000 a year over newer therapies.

Caffeine is one of the metabolites of theophylline, and has similar, though weaker, bronchodilator action. Many a time a midnight asthma attack has been ameliorated with a little coffee. This does not mean you shouldn't have a rescue inhaler on hand. But if you're stuck overnight in an airport and don't have one with you, load up on caffeine until you can find your medicine. (And if you're really in trouble, ask for help or call 911.)

Lastly, get rid of the guinea pig, or at least, keep it outside.

Web sites with money-saving offers include:

www.advair.com

www.asmanex.com

www.maxairautohalercoupon.com

www.mysymbicort.com

www.proairhfa.com

www.proventilhfa.com

www.singulair.com

www.ventolinhfa.com

34. Depression: Spend less and stay happy

Family doctors treat depression on a daily basis. For most people referral to a psychiatrist or psychologist is not necessary, and seeing your family doctor is usually less expensive.

However, counseling often does help and most insurance plans offer at least limited coverage for counseling services. (As of January 1, 2010, the federal Mental Health Parity and Addiction Act requires group insurance plans for companies of 50 or more employees to provide mental health benefits, including counseling, on a par with coverage for physical illnesses.)

If psychiatric or psychological counseling is not covered but regular doctor visits are, ask your family doctor to consider offering counseling herself. Your local community, school, university, employer, or church may offer counseling services at a reduced rate as well.

Another resource is your local community health center, health department, or community mental health center, which may have an income-based sliding-fee scale for treatment, including medication. Federally funded health centers throughout the United States offer discounted services for low-income individuals. Find one in your state at: www.findahealthcenter .hrsa.gov/Search_HCC_byCounty.aspx.

Simply talking about how you feel is important. If you don't want to go to counseling, find a trusted friend or family member willing to share your concerns. They needn't have an answer for you—they only need to listen. Also, find something you enjoy to take your mind off your own unhappiness. Although it's difficult when you're depressed, doing something good for others helps take the focus off your own problems and increases your self-worth.

Over the years I've found the most useful advice I can offer depressed patients is the assurance that they will, indeed, feel better. The dark days won't last forever. There is hope for a brighter future.

In recent years so many antidepressants have become available in generic form that it's usually possible to find a cost-effective medication to treat depression. Generics for Prozac, Paxil, and Celexa (selective serotonin reuptake inhibitors, SSRIs) are now on the $4 list (see #16), as are several older antidepressants, including amitriptyline, doxepin, nortriptyline, and trazodone. Buspirone (generic Buspar), lithium, and several major tranquilizers are on the $4 list as well.

If your doctor prescribes a brand-name medication, ask for samples (see #17) or discuss the possibility of using a different medication. Remind your doctor if you're self-pay, and bring a copy of your formulary and/or $4 list with you. Patient assistance programs, such as the Together Rx Access program (www.togetherrxaccess.com, see #18), are an additional option.

Web sites with discounts or coupons:

www.cymbalta.com

www.effexorxr.com

www.pristiq.com

Whatever you and your doctor decide, take your medicine as prescribed and follow up with your doctor. It helps to get feedback on your progress. If you have side effects, call your physician before discontinuing the medication, as sometimes this triggers withdrawal-like symptoms. Eventually you will feel better, so don't give up. Someone does care about you.

35. Diabetes: Sweet deals to keep your sugar under control

You diet and exercise and still your blood sugar is too high. Your doctor says it's time to start medication but you worry about the cost.

The cost of medication is only one of the expenses diabetics face. Frequent doctor visits, periodic lab work, and home blood sugar monitoring also factor into the equation. The most expensive aspect of diabetic treatment is management of long-term side effects, including heart and kidney disease.

In modern medicine the trend is to use the latest and theoretically "best" treatments. But new usually means expensive, and sometimes means doctors lack sufficient information regarding long-term administration.

The newer diabetic medications offer the potential advantage of longer-term glucose control, delaying the need for additional pills or insulin. Theoretically this would also translate into fewer complications of diabetes, but that is not necessarily true in all individuals.

If you can't afford to buy your medications, they won't

help at all. With newer drugs running $100, $200, or more a month, self-pay patients need an effective, economical regimen to manage their disease. Even insured patients may have $50 co-pays on brand-name drugs, which can add up to thousands of dollars a year.

One place to start is the $4 list (see #16). Unless your doctor insists on one of the newer medications, he or she will probably initiate treatment with metformin. Both the immediate and extended-release forms are now available for $4 a month. Metformin has the advantages of not causing weight gain and rarely causing hypoglycemia (low blood sugar). The disadvantage is that some patients suffer intestinal side effects, making it difficult to tolerate the drug. However, starting at a low dose and gradually increasing the medication to a therapeutic level allows most patients to tolerate metformin. For diabetics on metformin alone, home blood sugar monitoring is optional (see below).

Prior to the release of glitazone drugs (Actos, Avandia), the sulfonylurea drugs were the standard of care and are still appropriate for many patients. The older medication chlorpropamide and the newer sulfonylureas—glimepiride, glipizide, and glyburide—are all on the $4 list. This class of drugs has a greater potential to cause low blood sugar as well as weight gain but rarely produces stomach upset. Many patients take both metformin and a sulfonylurea drug, an affordable combination.

The cost of medication alone can run thousands of dollars a year. Your doctor may be only vaguely aware of drug prices, so feel free to help educate him or her. Whereas pharmaceutical representatives often inform doctors regarding which insurance plans cover the drugs they're promoting, they rarely mention retail pricing unless specifically asked.

Approximate Monthly Pricing for Other Diabetic Medications	
Actos and ActoPlus	$120–$245
Avandia and Avandamet	$180–$266
Byetta (1 pen)	$270
Glyset	$100–$120
Humalog (1 vial)	$120
Humulin (1 vial)	$62
Januvia	$210
Lantus	$110
Levemir	$110
Novolin	$73
NovoLog	$118
Onglyza	$200
Prandin, PrandiMet	$72
Precose	$80–$100
Starlix	$65
Symlin (1 vial)	$225
Insulin needles run $20–$40 per box of 100	
Insulin "pens" may add additional expense	

For those patients who require but cannot afford the above drugs, patient assistance programs are helpful (see #18). The Together Rx Access program (www.togetherrxaccess.com,

1-800-444-4106) offers discounts on over 300 brand-name prescription medicines. If you have no prescription drug coverage, you are not eligible for Medicare, and your income is less than $45,000 for a single person ($90,000 for a family of four), you are eligible for the card.

Covered diabetic medications and blood sugar testing products include:

- Actos products
- Avandia products
- FreeStyle blood glucose testing products
- Glucotrol
- Glynase
- Glyset
- One Touch blood glucose testing products
- Precision blood glucose testing products
- Starlix

Many Medicare patients are eligible to receive free insulin and blood sugar testing supplies through local and mail-away pharmacies.

In addition to medication to lower your blood sugar, your doctor will likely suggest an ACE (angiotensin-converting enzyme) inhibitor to protect your kidneys from the effects of high blood sugar. Lisinopril, benazepril, captopril, and enalapril are all on the $4 list. These drugs are also used for high blood pressure and heart failure, so you may be able to reap a double benefit. If you cannot tolerate an ACE inhibitor (due to cough or other side effect), your doctor may prescribe an ARB (angiotensin receptor blocker). By mid-2010 the first generic ARB will be available.

Home blood sugar testing adds a significant expense to diabetic care but may not be necessary, especially if your sugar is well controlled using acarbose and/or metformin alone. Ask your doctor whether you need to test, and if so, how often. Also ask what the goal of doing so is. There is little point in testing yourself if the results do not impact your treatment plan. Home glucose testing can be useful in assessing compliance, detecting patterns of high or low blood sugars, and correlating symptoms with blood glucose levels. But if the number is merely recorded and ignored, it only adds an additional level of expense.

If you will be doing home blood sugar testing, check with your insurance company regarding which monitor they prefer. Testing strips are like printer ink cartridges: the supplies may cost more than the machine itself, from $50 to $140 per hundred strips. Also see the list on page 86 for products on the Together Rx Access program.

Testing your hemoglobin A1C (average blood sugar) every four to six months instead of every three may save you $50–$100 a year. If your diabetes is well controlled, ask your doctor if this is appropriate for you.

Diabetics should also have an annual EKG, a urinalysis, an eye exam (see #4), and be tested for cholesterol (see #39).

Web sites with coupons for diabetic drugs:

www.actos.com

www.avandia.com

www.januvia.com

www.onglyza.com

---

36. Enlarged prostate: Sweet dreams and sleep soundly

It's *not* normal to wake up three times a night to urinate.

As men age, the prostate enlarges—just like the ears. Prostatic enlargement may "squeeze" the urethra (the tube draining the bladder), causing frequent urination (both day and night), slower urine stream, and trouble initiating urination or dribbling afterward.

Similar symptoms may be caused by low-grade prostate or urine infection as well (or occasionally prostate cancer), so see your doctor and have your urine checked for a definitive diagnosis. Symptoms of acute or chronic prostatitis are often relieved with a $4 antibiotic. Of course, a person can have both a prostate infection and an enlarged prostate, sometimes making it difficult to distinguish the two.

For an enlarged prostate, there are two modes of treatment: shrink the prostate (with medicine or surgery) or relax the pressure from the prostate on the urethra, or both.

The antiandrogen drugs, which partially block the effect of male hormones on the prostate, help shrink the prostate and relieve symptoms in about 50 percent of patients. Medication takes at least four to six weeks to begin working, and may take six months to reach full effect. Of the antiandrogens, finasteride (brand name Proscar) now comes in generic, currently about $70 a month versus $110 for brand name. A newer medication, dutasteride (Avodart), may work better in some patients. It costs a little more ($125 a month) but your doctor may have a coupon available, or check www .avodart.com.

Saw palmetto is an over-the-counter herb that relieves symptoms in about 50 percent of men who take it at the recommended dose of 100 to 400 milligrams twice a day. It may work as well as prescription medication and costs only $10–$20 a month. Many doctors prescribe saw palmetto in place of the antiandrogen drugs.

Relaxing the pressure on the urethra (using an alpha-blocker) produces quicker results than shrinking the prostate, often within days to weeks of beginning therapy. Due to the rapid relief of symptoms and lower cost, doctors often use alpha-blockers for initial treatment. Three of these medications—doxazosin (Cardura), prazosin (Minipres), and terazosin (Hytrin)—are also used for high blood pressure, with generic versions available on the $4 list (see #16).

A newer alpha-blocker, Flomax, helps relax the prostate but does not lower blood pressure. Early in 2010 it became available in a generic form as well, at a savings of 20–30 percent over name-brand medication (but still over $100 a month). The cost is likely to drop further as more generic manufacturers provide additional competition. Your doctor may still have a coupon for brand name Flomax, but nearly every time a drug goes generic, coupon programs are discontinued. Rapaflo (silodosin) is another new brand-name alpha-blocker, currently priced about the same as generic Flomax ($120 a month). The manufacturer offers a coupon toward your co-pay on a *different* drug if Rapaflo is ineffective in treating your symptoms.

Both the antiandrogens and saw palmetto can be combined with the alpha-blockers if necessary. Surgery remains an option for advanced or resistant cases. For mild cases, some men decline treatment altogether, preferring to live with the symptoms. Discuss this option with your doctor before discontinuing any medication. At times the problem may be more advanced than you know, preventing the bladder from emptying completely, thereby putting back-pressure on the kidneys, which may result in serious complications.

For more information about benign prostatic enlargement, visit www.mayoclinic.com/health/prostate-gland -enlargement/DS00027.

37. GERD and gastritis: Analyze your annoying acid

GERD, gastritis, ulcers, hiatal hernia: what's the difference and what does it matter?

Each of these conditions is in some way related to a stomach acid condition. Because each may produce the same symptoms and at times respond to the same treatment, it's often difficult to tell the difference.

GERD, also known as gastroesophageal reflux disease, is a condition where too much stomach acid refluxes upward from the stomach into the esophagus. In general, the stomach is designed to tolerate hydrochloric acid whereas the esophagus is not. Splashing acid up your esophagus repeatedly is much like pouring acid on your hand. After awhile it causes irritation, producing symptoms of burning and/or pain in the chest or upper abdomen. Sometimes reflux results in burping or regurgitation, or a cough, wheezing, or difficulty swallowing. We all have a little reflux, but the contractions of our esophagus as we swallow our saliva wash the acid back into the stomach.

Acid reflux is made worse by a variety of foods and behaviors. The cheapest answer is simple—behave yourself. Don't smoke. Don't drink. Don't worry. Don't exercise right after you eat. Don't eat late at night. Don't eat too much. Don't eat spicy foods, acidic foods (tomatoes, citrus), chocolate, coffee, caffeine, fried foods, and so forth—basically if it's tasty, don't eat it. Think of the money you'll save!

Also, beware of drugs such as aspirin, ibuprofen, naproxen, prednisone, and other steroids, all of which can make reflux worse.

If avoiding the above irritants doesn't resolve your symptoms, you may require medication. Medication is aimed at lessening the acid in your esophagus by either: neutralizing the acid with an antacid, making your stomach produce less acid, improving the contractions in your esophagus, or coating your esophagus.

For occasional symptoms, antacids (or even baking soda) are the quickest, cheapest treatment (5¢ for baking soda, $5 for Maalox or Rolaids).

For more persistent symptoms, acid reducers are commonly used (read #91 and #92 for a complete discussion). Generic H_2 inhibitors (Pepcid, Zantac, Tagamet) cost as little as $4 a month by prescription, but may cost more over the counter. OTC proton pump inhibitors (PPIs) run about $30 a month, but insured patients may actually pay less out of pocket for prescription medication, depending on your formulary and whether you can find a coupon to offset your co-pay. For cash-paying patients, the OTC PPIs (Prilosec and Prevacid) are your best bet.

Medication that helps clear stomach acid out of the esophagus more quickly is another approach. Generic metoclopramide is inexpensive (under $20), is available by prescription only, can be used daily or on an as-needed basis, and may be combined with an acid-reducing medication.

Lastly, simply put, sucralfate works by coating the esophagus. Generic sucralfate costs about $40 per 100, a hundred dollar savings over name brand.

In most patients GERD is a matter of comfort. But chronic exposure of the esophagus to acid can lead to scarring or even malignancy, so be sure to talk with your doctor if you have more than occasional symptoms.

Whereas GERD is a disorder of bodily function, a hiatal hernia is a structural abnormality. The stomach should reside within the abdominal cavity. However, sometimes the stomach "herniates" up through the diaphragm into the chest cavity.

Many patients have no symptoms whatsoever. (The diagnosis is sometimes made on a routine chest X-ray.) Other patients complain of a sense of fullness in the chest or abdomen, or discomfort with overeating. Some experience heartburn or reflux. A few patients undergo surgery to correct a hiatal hernia, but since GERD symptoms may persist even if the hernia is corrected, surgery is seldom recommended.

Gastritis is inflammation of the stomach lining. A short-lived episode may be due to a stomach virus, and requires no specific treatment. Sometimes a brief episode will set off a longer episode, which may respond to an acid-lowering medication or sucralfate. Like reflux, gastritis may be caused by anti-inflammatory medication such as aspirin, as well as alcohol or irritating foods.

However, gastritis may be a precursor to ulcer disease. Stomach ulcers and duodenal ulcers are both erosions. Severe erosion carries the risk of stomach bleeding or even perforation. Some, but not all, ulcers are caused by infection due to *Helicobacter pylori*. Abolishing the bacterial infection may actually cure an ulcer, although recurrence is possible. In addition to using one of the PPIs, your doctor will prescribe an antibiotic. If you are self-pay, request something from the $4 list.

Testing for the above conditions involves fluoroscopic X-rays or endoscopy, which runs hundreds to thousands of dollars. Specialists are more likely than primary care doctors to order these tests, so discuss the situation with your family doctor first. A therapeutic trial of medication is usually effective and much less expensive. The decision whether to obtain additional testing also depends on your age, your general health, and the circumstances surrounding your stomach problem. For example, if you're 35 years old and have stomach discomfort after taking ibuprofen for a sprained ankle, you probably don't need a scope—just lay off the ibuprofen. If you're 70 years old and are experiencing heartburn and weight loss, you need a thorough evaluation.

Offers on Prescription PPIs

www.aciphex.com or call 1-800-952-0400

www.dexilant.com

www.prevacid24HR.com or call 1-800-452-0051

www.prilosecotc.com

www.purplepill.com

Protonix is available through the Wyeth Patient Assistance Program at 1-800-568-9938 or www.wyeth.com/contact?rid=/wyeth_html/home/shared/footer/Patient/contact_patient_assist.html. Pantoprazole is also available generic.

---

38. High blood pressure: Take the tension out of hypertension

Is your blood pressure high enough without worrying about the cost of your medicine?

Although some people can lower their blood pressure to normal levels through diet, weight loss, and exercise, the majority will need at least one medication, and many will need two or more.

The Joint National Committee on Prevention, Detection, Evaluation, and Treatment of High Blood Pressure continues to recommend inexpensive diuretics (water pills) as first-line treatment for high blood pressure. The definition of high blood pressure is 140/90 or greater, with levels of 120–139/80–89 considered prehypertension.

Of the various types of water pills, thiazide-type diuretics are used most commonly for hypertension. Luckily these are dirt cheap. Several first-line beta-blockers are on the $4 list as well (see #16), including atenolol, metoprolol, nadolol, and pindolol. Each of these is the short-acting version of the drug and may need to be taken twice a day. The trade-off for the greater convenience of once-a-day medication is higher price. For example, 24-hour metoprolol costs $35 to $70 a month, whereas the equivalent dose of a 12-hour twice a day pill is $4 to $15.

Some patients cannot tolerate water pills or beta-blockers. Others experience insufficient lowering of their blood pressure with these medications. If so, branching out to other classes of medication is the next move. The $4 list includes several angiotensin-converting enzyme (ACE) inhibitors. These are a great choice for diabetic patients, who should be on them anyway, to protect the kidneys from the effect of high blood sugar.

Occasionally, ACE inhibitors cause a cough or other side effect. If so, your doctor will probably prescribe an ARB (angiotensin receptor blocker) instead. Because these drugs are newer than the ACE inhibitors, most are not available in a generic version. However, 2010 marks the expiration of Merck's patent on Cozaar, so generic losartan should be available shortly. What this will do is push formularies to cover this generic over the other brand-name ARBs (Atacand, Avapro, Benicar, Diovan, Micardis, and Teveten). For insured patients, switching to generic losartan may lower your co-pay. For cash-paying patients, the generic should be priced at least 10 percent below brand-name Cozaar, and should drop further over the next year or so. If you need an ARB that is not covered, check into the patient assistance programs.

A fifth class of medications, the alpha-blockers (doxazosin, prazosin, and terazosin), are all on the $4 list. Lastly, several calcium channel blockers come in generic forms for $20 to $40 a month.

With so many choices, surely your doctor can find something appropriate for your needs.

In addition to the cost of medication, patients with high blood pressure need to consider the cost of office visits and laboratory testing. Some doctors require an annual EKG, but self-pay patients may want to ask if less frequent testing is appropriate. One drawback to the use of inexpensive diuretics is the need for periodic blood tests to monitor sodium, potassium, and kidney function. It may actually cost less to use a slightly more expensive drug that does not require blood monitoring.

Patients who get serious about their condition may be

able to avoid medication altogether. Eliminating excess salt and calories from the diet can make a huge difference. Likewise, regular exercise and avoidance of tobacco help lower the blood pressure. Weight loss would help nearly all hypertensive patients. These same measures often lower blood sugar and cholesterol as well, further reducing cardiovascular risk.

Home blood pressure monitoring is not usually necessary. Only buy a monitor if your doctor thinks it will enhance your treatment plan.

With high blood pressure so common, the treatment of hypertension often affords the opportunity to alleviate two problems with one medication. If you have any of the following in addition to high blood pressure, ask your doctor about using a single medication to alleviate both conditions:

- Angina (beta-blockers, calcium channel blockers)
- Anxiety, stage fright, or tremor (beta-blockers, clonidine)
- Atrial fibrillation (beta-blockers, calcium-channel blockers)
- Benign prostatic hypertrophy (alpha-blockers)
- Congestive heart failure (ACE inhibitors)
- Diabetes (ACE inhibitors, ARBs)
- Diarrhea (verapamil or other nondihydropyridine calcium channel blockers)
- Insomnia (clonidine)
- Migraines or other headaches (beta-blockers, calcium channel blockers, and others)

- Palpitations or irregular heartbeat (beta-blockers, calcium channel blockers)
- Raynaud's syndrome (dihydropyridine calcium channel blockers)
- Swelling (diuretics, ACE inhibitors)

39. High cholesterol: Fatten your wallet, not your blood

The reason to treat high cholesterol is to decrease the risk for cardiovascular disease, that is, heart attacks and strokes.

Serum cholesterol levels may be elevated based on diet, genetics, or both. People with high cholesterol due to diet sometimes require no medication. I've had patients lower their total cholesterol by 30, 60, even 100 points simply by avoiding fats in their diet.

Should you have your cholesterol checked? The U.S. Preventive Services Task Force recommends screening all men age 35 and older for high cholesterol, and men age 20 and older at increased risk of heart disease (tobacco use, diabetes, high blood pressure, obesity, those with a family history of heart disease or high cholesterol). Women over age 20 with risk factors should also be screened, though there are no specific recommendations for low-risk women. Spend a few minutes discussing these recommendations with your doctor at your next visit.

Screening involves blood testing. For ways to save money on cholesterol tests, see #53, 54, 55, 57, and 79. Although a full cholesterol panel runs $75 to $150, you may be able to find testing for free or reduced cost.

Most patients with elevated total or LDL cholesterol levels are advised to follow a low-fat, low-cholesterol diet. Patients with high HDL levels (the "good" cholesterol) may not need to do so. Niacin, a vitamin, helps to increase HDL levels and is available over the counter for about $20 a month. Please read the label regarding dosage and flushing before using niacin.

The typical American diet is too high in fat and cholesterol. Aim for less than 200 milligrams of cholesterol daily with under 30 percent of your calories from fat, and under 7 percent of your calories from saturated fat. Changing your diet is cheaper than taking medication. For a good discussion, visit the Cholesterol Management Guide at www.webmd.com.

Only one prescription medication works by blocking the absorption of dietary cholesterol. Zetia (ezetimibe) costs about $120 a month and does not come in generic. If your doctor feels this is the best medication for you and cost is a concern, visit the Merck/Schering Plough patient assistance Web site at www.msppharma.com/msp_jv/msppharma/patient_assist/index.jsp or call 1-800-347-7503. Vytorin, a combination of Zetia and simvastatin, is also covered under this program.

Patients who have the genetic disposition to excess cholesterol production usually need a "statin" to counter this inherited trait. The most powerful (and most expensive) of the statins are Crestor and Lipitor, both of which are currently available by brand name only. The patent on Lipitor expires within the next year, however, at which time generic atorvastatin will become available. Fortunately, both Crestor and Lipitor offer flat pricing. The highest dose pills may be split in half (or even quarters), thereby cutting your cost by 50 (or even 75) percent (see #14).

If your cholesterol isn't sky high you can probably be treated with one of the generic equivalents for Zocor, Pravachol, or Mevacor. All three are on certain $4 lists in at least one strength, and each of them may be split as well (see #14 and #16).

High cholesterol isn't the whole story on heart disease. Some patients with normal cholesterol will suffer heart at-

---

Useful Web sites with money-saving offers:

www.astrazeneca-us.com offers help for uninsured patients requiring Crestor

www.crestor.com

www.lipitor.com

www.pfizerhelpfulanswers.com offers help for uninsured patients requiring Lipitor, or call 1-866-706-2400

www.trilipix.com

www.zetia.com offers a link to the patient assistance program for Merck/Schering-Plough for Zetia or Vytorin, or call 1-800-347-7503 tacks. Medical science continues to search for better answers as to who is at greatest risk. For now, it's a good idea to limit *all* your risk factors—don't smoke, maintain a good weight, watch your diet, and choose your parents carefully.

40. Obesity: Sweet savings to shrink your surplus

Eat less. OK, that's simplistic (however accurate).

But seriously, SAVE YOUR MONEY AND SKIP THE OTC MEDICATIONS. They rarely work. With the exception of orlistat, very few OTC products have scientific proof of effectiveness.

As for prescription medications, at present there are only a few with FDA approval for weight loss. After the Redux scare of a decade ago, governmental regulation of weight-loss medications has tightened. Only phentermine (Adipex-P), sibutramine (Meridia), and orlistat (Xenical, Alli) are currently in common use for weight loss, and all but Alli are by prescription.

Of these, phentermine and sibutramine are appetite suppressants, whereas orlistat blocks about a third of dietary fat from being absorbed. Phentermine is indicated for short-term use only. Sibutramine is indicated for weight loss or to help maintain weight loss, for up to two years. Some physicians refuse to prescribe either of these medications due to concerns with abuse, long-term effectiveness, or the belief that patients should not rely on medication for weight loss.

Appetite suppressants work by altering the brain chemicals that control appetite, a complex mechanism. Suppressing one chemical may lead to an increase in another, which is why the medications don't continue to work with prolonged administration, and perhaps why many people gain weight after discontinuing the medication. Overall, the appetite mechanism is wonderfully designed and present throughout the animal kingdom. Imagine if your dog had to calculate how many calories it needed. But both humans and animals are prone to weight gain when given unrestricted access to high-calorie food in conjunction with inadequate exercise.

Regarding exercise, it takes a half hour of walking to consume 100–250 calories, depending on speed. Since a pound of fat contains 3,500 calories, in order to lose one pound a week, you will need to consume 500 calories per day less, or exercise 500 calories per day more (an hour or more of walking daily).

Another interesting note: most of the calories we burn are used to keep our bodies warm. Exercise consumes 25 percent or less for people of average activity. Some medications that cause weight gain (e.g., Zyprexa) may actually do so by setting our internal thermostat lower, thus requiring fewer calories to fuel our system.

Back to the medications: appetite suppressants are effective, at least in the short-term. They work by far the best the first time the body is exposed to them. If your doctor prescribes an appetite suppressant, take advantage of your decreased appetite while you can. Get your stomach and body accustomed to smaller meals. Start an exercise program. Understand that these medications are intended to be an adjunct to lifestyle changes within your control. Only phentermine comes in a generic version, at about $20 a month. Some states limit use of phentermine to three months. Because phentermine has mild stimulant properties, it is not advisable in patients with high blood pressure, heart disease, anxiety, or certain other chronic diseases. In a young, otherwise healthy adult, however, it can help patients lose up to 10 pounds a month for a few months.

Meridia (sibutramine) is available by brand name only and runs over $100 monthly. In the average patient, Meridia suppresses the appetite less strongly than does phentermine but is approved for maintaining weight loss as well as for losing weight. It, too, has potential side effects, including headaches, dry mouth, and blood pressure elevation. The Together Rx Access program offers a discount on Meridia for uninsured, non-Medicare patients who meet their income guidelines (under $60,000 yearly for a family of two). Call 1-800-444-4106 or visit www.togetherrxaccess.com. Avoid online offers for generic Meridia, which does not exist in the United States.

In Ohio (and elsewhere) monthly physician visits are required with both phentermine and Meridia. Some insurance plans cover these medications but may require preauthorization or a letter from your doctor verifying your weight, BMI (body mass index), and unsuccessful attempts at weight loss. Although office visits and medication are costly, investing in yourself and your future is important as well. Talk to your doctor about how best to meet your needs.

As for orlistat, a fat-blocker (Xenical, Alli), read #95 for a complete discussion.

Lastly, regarding weight-loss surgery, some insurance will pay the $10,000 to $40,000 fee if you meet certain criteria, but preauthorization is *always* required. For patients needing to lose 100 pounds or more, especially for those with additional medical problems, bariatric surgery is an option.

Like I said at the beginning, eat less—it's cheaper.

CHAPTER FIVE

Save Money on Acute Illness

41. Athlete's foot and other foot fungi

If you have sweaty, stinky, smelly feet—with a rash and maybe itching—odds are good it's athlete's foot. Sweaty feet are a breeding ground for fungus.

Foot fungus comes in two main varieties. The moist, itchy, smelly kind is more common in younger individuals with sweaty feet. It commonly presents between or under the toes and is sometimes mistaken for poison ivy. A picture atlas of athlete's foot and other common skin conditions is available online at www.dermatlas.com/derm.

It's very difficult to cure this foot infection when your feet (or shoes) stay wet. Wear clean, dry, white socks, let your feet "breathe," and discard those smelly sneakers. Buy a new pair for 10 bucks and wear them until your feet are well. Then throw them out and get a good pair.

The dry, scaly variety commonly involves the soles and sides of the feet in a "moccasin" pattern and is more common in older patients. It is often mistaken for dry skin and may persist unrecognized for years. Sometimes it is accompanied by fungal infection of the toenails, which may appear thickened, yellow, and somewhat brittle. Occasionally, this type of fungal infection affects the hands as well.

If you're sure you have athlete's foot, save a trip to the doctor and treat yourself. Excellent antifungal medications are available over the counter, both brand name (Tinactin, Lotrimin AF, and Lamisil) or generics of the same for as little as $5 to $15. Visit your local pharmacy for any of these products. One "trick" to effective use: apply the cream *daily* until the rash is entirely gone, then *continue* using the product *another* week or two. Recurrence is likely if even microscopic levels of the fungus remain. At least half the patients I see for athlete's foot have already tried the correct medicine but did not use it long enough and did not discard their infected shoes. You must use the antifungal medicine *at least* two weeks, often three or four, to insure a complete cure.

If the OTC preparations have not helped *at all* by a week or two, please do consult your doctor, especially if things are getting worse. What appears to be athlete's foot may be something else entirely. Diabetics, patients with poor circulation, psoriasis, swelling, or nail fungus may have particular problems. Sometimes contact dermatitis will masquerade as athlete's foot, and occasionally a bacterial infection will set in.

But assuming it is merely persistent athlete's foot and the creams aren't working, ask your doctor about two oral antifungal agents that now come in generic forms. Once costing hundreds of dollars, fluconazole and terbinafine are available on some $4 lists (see #16), but the amount and dosage may vary from store to store. The pills are more effective than the creams and may end up costing less as well. Check a few $4 lists online (see appendix 4) before visiting your physician. Doctors appreciate patients who do their homework, and it doesn't save you money when a doctor has to look up something for you that you could do yourself.

If the rash is especially inflamed (red) or itchy, a little OTC hydrocortisone cream can be added to any of the above regimens. Stronger steroid creams (also on the $4 list) are sometimes prescribed and do *appear* to work better, though may actually slow clearing of the infection. They offer rapid relief from itching and redness but can suppress your own healing process. Also, since they give the illusion of healing, patients stop using the medication too soon, allowing the infection to persist.

Fluconazole and terbinafine are effective for fungus of the toenails as well but must be used for *much* longer periods, usually several months—and even then they don't always work. If your toenails are infected with fungus but are not bothering you, you can save money by simply leaving them alone. *No* over-the-counter medicine is effective, so don't waste your money.

42. Broken toes and painful pinkies

Don't swear at the bedpost. If you've stubbed your toe hard enough to make you curse, you may well have broken it. Other ways to break a toe include:

- Being stepped on by a horse or high heels
- Kicking a ball or an unfortunate teammate

- Dropping a car battery or computer on your foot
- Hitting your toe with a golf club or baseball bat
- Suffering a car, motorcycle, or bicycle accident

Medically speaking, there's a difference between the little toes and the big toe. The big toe helps maintain balance, and of course the bones are bigger. *If you think you've broken your big toe, see your doctor.*

The smaller toes are less crucial. Unless the toe is visibly deformed or cut open, a fracture is managed the same as a bad bruise. The bones are tiny and heal without surgery or casting. Wearing a flat-bottom shoe that prevents movement of the toe joints may lessen the discomfort, as may rest, ice, elevation, and OTC anti-inflammatory medicines or acetaminophen. Taping the injured toe to the adjacent uninjured digit provides a handy splint.

If you're young and healthy and your toe looks a little swollen and/or bruised, there's no urgency to seek medical attention. But even if you're healthy, if your toe is very deformed or if the pain extends up into your foot, or if you have an open wound, you should see your doctor. You may also need to see your doctor if you need time off work from a physically demanding job.

If you're diabetic, have poor circulation, have no clear-cut history of injury, or are in general poor health, please see your doctor. Other conditions such as gout, arthritis, cancer, and infection sometimes masquerade as a fracture.

Regarding X-rays, a simple toe fracture with a clear-cut history of trauma does not necessarily require an X-ray. But if you go to an urgent care center or emergency room with an injured toe, odds are you'll have an X-ray. If you go to your family doctor, especially if your doctor does not have X-ray equipment on site, you're much less likely to incur the expense of X-rays. Ask your doctor if you truly need an X-ray—often they're done more to make a patient happy than because a doctor thinks the procedure is mandatory.

Other common causes of painful toes include ingrown nails, Raynaud's phenomenon, subungual hematoma, bunions, hammertoes, and metatarsalgia.

For ingrown nails, prevention is ideal. Make sure you cut your nails such that sharp corners cannot pierce your skin. However, genetic predisposition can be blamed for many cases of ingrown toenails. The nail is shaped such that the edges rather than the end of the nail grow too far into your skin, causing irritation and sometimes infection. Avoiding undue pressure on the nail, for example, by wearing properly fitted shoes, helps prevent recurrences. Occasionally, an infected nail can be permanently cured with a $4 antibiotic (and good shoes). However, the swelling and irritation tend to recur, eventually requiring excision of the lateral portion of the nail. Some doctors advise this minor surgery for the first occurrence, to save pain, time, and aggravation on future recurrences.

Raynaud's phenomenon is a circulatory condition that can make the toes (or fingers) turn red, white, or blue when exposed to cold. The most important thing is to keep your hands and feet warm using socks, gloves, and/or hand and foot warmers. Keeping the center of your body warm—your chest and abdomen—helps as well, because this allows your body to shunt more blood to your extremities. Most people require no medication, though some patients do well with certain blood pressure medications that dilate the blood vessels. Keeping yourself warm during the winter months can save money on medicine and doctor visits.

A subungual hematoma is a collection of blood underneath the toenail or fingernail. Unlike a bruise, where the blood soaks into the surrounding tissue like a sponge, with a hematoma the blood forms a pool, more like a water balloon. If you've dropped a hammer on your toe and developed a painful black spot underneath the nail you have two options: live with it (for free) or consider relieving the pressure caused by the trapped blood. Untreated, the pain usually resolves within a few days. Keep in mind if the toe itself is painful, not just the nail, you may have fractured your toe (see page 107). Also, if you are diabetic or have poor circulation, you should probably see your doctor rather than treat yourself at home. For healthy individuals, relieving the pressure oneself is an option—for the cost of a paper clip. I am not necessarily recommending you do this yourself, but if you're stuck in Antarctica, it is an option. For a good video of how a doctor would treat this condition go to: www.you tube.com/watch?v=x7yNSVDg_l4.

Bunions and hammer toes are deformities of the toe joints. Although some patients undergo surgery for these conditions, having your shoes sized professionally may be all that's required to relieve the discomfort. Though you may have worn a size 8A in high school, a 9C may fit you now. A $200 pair of shoes might save you thousands on toe surgery or diabetic foot ulcer treatment. If your foot is misshapen, ask about stretching your shoe in the appropriate area. For diabetics at risk of foot ulcers, Medicare (and sometimes private insurance) will pay for diabetic shoes.

Metatarsalgia simply means pain across the bottom of your foot at the base of the toes, where the foot bones meet the toes bones. If your doctor has diagnosed this condition, or if you'd like to try treating yourself before consulting a doctor, in addition to properly fitting shoes, a metatarsal pad may relieve your symptoms. Metatarsal pads are available without a prescription from shoe stores, orthopedic supply stores, and many online vendors for under $20. For an excellent discussion of metatarsalgia visit the Mayo Clinic's Web site at: www.mayoclinic.com/health/metatarsalgia/DS00496.

43. Laryngitis and pharyngitis (sore throat)

Laryngitis—inflammation of the larynx—produces hoarseness, or a "lost" voice. Swelling of the vocal cords may make it difficult to talk above a whisper, or in lesser cases just make your voice a little gruff or lower pitched than usual.

The most common cause of laryngitis is a viral infection, such as a cold or viral pharyngitis. Laryngitis is fairly uncommon with bacterial infections, particularly strep throat. If you have a mild sore throat and your voice is hoarse, odds are it isn't strep.

Losing your voice as part of a cold is not really a reason to see your doctor—more of a reason not to. Stay home and save the cost of an office visit, a strep test, and an antibiotic—you should be well in a few days. Resting the voice allows the vocal cords to heal. Continued use of the voice will only cause the swelling to persist. Hot tea or Tylenol may soothe the throat, and a decongestant may decrease swelling a bit.

But the most helpful remedy is *don't talk*.

Sometimes persistent coughing may cause hoarseness. Use an over-the-counter cough suppressant (dextromethorphan) or an antihistamine such as diphenhydramine if drainage is causing the cough. See your doctor if the cough persists or is accompanied by worsening symptoms or shortness of breath.

Reasons to see a doctor for a hoarse voice:

- Work that involves speaking and therefore the need for a medical excuse.
- Hoarseness that persists beyond a week or two, especially if not accompanied by a cold, and especially if you're a smoker—vocal cord tumors may cause hoarseness.
- Hoarseness accompanied by persistent heartburn—acid reflux may damage the vocal cords and cause hoarseness.
- Hoarseness along with other respiratory symptoms that persist beyond a week or two—occasionally antibiotics do help.
- Hoarseness accompanied by difficulty swallowing—neurologic problems such as a stroke may cause this combination.
- Hoarseness accompanied by shortness of breath—*see your doctor right away*. Children especially may have

swelling in the trachea or epiglottis that can close off the airway quite suddenly.

Pharyngitis is inflammation of the throat (pharynx). Looking in a mirror you can see the upper pharynx and tonsils at the back of your mouth, behind the tongue. The larynx, discussed earlier, lies below the pharynx, farther down the neck.

Pharyngitis often causes the sensation of a sore throat—but not always. Interestingly, some patients with terrible-looking throats experience very little discomfort. Other patients whose throats appear normal complain of significant pain. Some people experience throat pain as ear pain or vice versa. The source of the pain can also be from swelling of the glands in the neck rather than the throat itself.

The general rule for pharyngitis is: if it's not strep, you don't need an antibiotic—at least not most of the time. However, even with strep throat the reason for antibiotic treatment has little to do with making your throat feel better. Rather, the antibiotics are to prevent rheumatic fever or heart disease, which can cause serious illness or damage your heart valves.

That said, how's a person to know what is and isn't strep without seeing a doctor?

Common causes of sore throat are:

- Viral pharyngitis (including "mono")
- Upper respiratory infection (colds)
- Strep throat (group A streptococcal infection)

Of these, only strep throat requires an antibiotic. Any other medication that your doctor prescribes is for symptom relief only rather than to cure the infection. An exception to this rule is a prolonged cold that seems to be getting worse instead of better, indicating the possibility of a secondary bacterial infection that may resolve more quickly with an antibiotic. Not all prolonged sore throats require an antibiotic, however. Especially in a teenager, a prolonged sore throat suggests the possibility of infectious mononucleosis, another virus. Doctors don't usually test for this infection early on since mononucleosis ("mono") often resolves in a week or two.

You can save money on sore throats by:

- Not seeing your doctor unnecessarily
- Not having a strep test unless needed
- Having only one strep test instead of two
- Not taking an antibiotic unnecessarily

You probably don't have strep throat if you:

- Have laryngitis (hoarseness)
- Have a cough
- Don't have a fever or feel especially ill
- Have drainage causing your sore throat

With the above symptoms, you can wait a few days and see how things go.

Strep throat is more likely with:

- A high fever
- A severe sore throat
- "Pus" on the tonsils
- Bad breath, nausea, or abdominal pain
- Red spots on the palate (top of the mouth)
- A faintly pink, fine, "sandpapery" rash

Consult your doctor if you have these symptoms. Ask if you need a strep test. (For a discussion of how to save money on strep tests, read #59.) If your doctor diagnoses strep throat, ask for a $4 antibiotic, which may be free at some pharmacies (Giant Eagle, Publix, Meijer, Stop & Shop, and others) during the cold and flu season.

44. Metal allergy (delayed hypersensitivity reaction): Infected earrings

Metal allergy is what causes most so-called pierced-ear infections. Many earrings contain nickel, a metal that causes skin sensitization.

But I've worn those earrings before and they never bothered me, you say.

Nickel allergy has what's called a sensitization phase and an elicitation phase. In the first phase your skin comes in contact with the metal but does not react. Eventually though, with repeat exposure, your skin becomes sensitized and begins to show signs of allergic irritation. In and around the area of contact your skin may be quite itchy and appear red, blistered, and scaly or cracked, and may ooze a clear yellow (serous) fluid.

And though earrings are a common source of nickel exposure, rings, necklaces, bracelets, belt buckles, and snaps can cause the problem as well.

The solution to nickel allergy is to avoid contact with nickel. Save money on a doctor's appointment by trying these at-home remedies.

First and primary, avoid *all* contact with nickel. Wear only fine gold earrings or other nickel-free earrings. If you don't keep an earring in the piercing site it is quite likely to grow over as the skin inflammation heals. Apply over-the-counter 1 percent hydrocortisone cream or ointment to the inflamed area. This, in conjunction with nickel avoidance and your own immune system, will resolve most cases.

If the crustiness of the ears does not resolve with the above measures, adding over-the-counter bacitracin antibiotic ointment may help. Certainly any open sore including those from nickel allergy can become infected. But one thing you don't want to do is apply triple antibiotic ointment to open, oozing sores. The neomycin in the preparation may cause the same allergic problem that nickel does.

If you're not sure if your jewelry contains nickel, you may want to test it. Athena Allergy offers the Nickel Solution Kit for about $20, available at www.natlallergy.com. The kit contains a solution to detect nickel, and also a preparation to apply to metal objects to protect skin from nickel exposure.

Often applying clear nail polish to jewelry can accomplish the same thing, but some people are sensitive or allergic to chemicals in nail polish. Remember that any product applied to metal to protect your skin will wear off with time and will require periodic reapplication.

It's far better to discontinue use of nickel-containing jewelry. No medication, not even prescription medication, can counteract ongoing exposure to the offending metal.

A severe case of metal allergy may require a visit to your doctor, who will likely prescribe a stronger prescription steroid cream for short-term use. Luckily, several are available for as little as $4. Occasionally, in addition to the allergic reaction, the earring site may become sufficiently infected to require oral antibiotics, but several of these are also on the $4 list at many pharmacies (see appendix 4). Hopefully, one case of metal allergy will be sufficient to convince you to follow the above guidelines.

45. Pink eye (conjunctivitis)

If I were in charge of the world, I wouldn't send kids home from school for a pink eye. For a goopy eye draining pus down the cheek, yes. But for an eye that's a little pink, no.

A pink eye is no worse than many other childhood illnesses. Lots of kids are at school with sore throats, influenza, impetigo, ringworm, pinworms, roundworms, scabies, bronchitis, and herpes, not to mention colds. And an eye that's somewhat pink is commonly a cold in the eye, not the dreaded "pink eye."

Many things can make an eye turn pink. Several years ago my niece's eye was a little itchy and red. She took a Visine bottle from the window sill to "get the red out." Unfortunately, it made her eye burn terribly and turn redder than ever. She ended up going to the ER where they diagnosed an allergic reaction to Visine.

This just goes to show that doctors aren't always right. When her brother came home later that day she learned he had put lighter fluid in the Visine bottle!

Other than caustic fluids, what can make your eyes turn pink? Colds and allergies are most common. Exposure to smoke, fumes, or other chemicals can cause a chemical conjunctivitis or reddening of the conjunctival membrane of the eye. Irritation from contact lenses, dry eyes, and trauma are additional causes. These require an antibiotic eye ointment only if the condition is severe, putting you at risk of secondary bacterial infection.

If you have a cold or a sore throat and your eye turns a little pink, it's usually a virus (viral conjunctivitis). You *are* contagious, same as a cold, but no worse. No antibiotics are needed. But that's not to say your doctor won't prescribe an eye antibiotic. By the time a parent has bothered to make an appointment, dragged her child to the doctor, waited an hour to spend five minutes with the doctor, she expects something—not to be told it's just a cold in the eye—and especially not when the school won't allow the child to return until the eye is better. Doctors do prescribe eye antibiotics even when they know it's a virus—except to their own kids. Prophylaxis against a secondary infection is often given as a reason, but this is unnecessary for the typical patient.

So if your kid's got a cold and his eye turns a little pink, save a trip to the doctor and the cost of medication by giving it a few days to resolve on its own. If your doctor does prescribe medication, ask for one on the $4 list—you shouldn't need an $80 eye drop.

However, bacterial conjunctivitis may be a sight-threatening condition and thus requires prompt medical attention. "*Eyes glued shut in the morning*" is an important indicator of bacterial infection. If you have abrupt onset of abundant, yellow-green eye discharge, especially without other symptoms of a cold, see your doctor right away.

Also see your doctor if your red eye is associated with pain or visual problems. These symptoms may indicate a corneal abrasion, glaucoma, or other serious inflammation.

Eye allergies to pollen, animals, and dust respond well to avoiding allergy triggers. Rinsing the offending allergen from the eyes is quite useful and may be all you need to do. Oral medicines that alleviate nasal allergies often relieve eye symptoms as well (see #31 for offers on allergy medications). Of the over-the-counter eye drops, those that contain naphazoline hydrochloride and/or pheniramine maleate are a good place to start and cost under $10. Another good choice is ketotifen (Zaditor). Once by prescription, it now is available OTC for about $15.

The prescription eye medications Patanol and Pataday (olopatadine) work wonderfully for many patients. But at over $100 a bottle, that can be a problem—especially when your daughter thinks they're just like Visine and uses the whole bottle in a weekend, like mine did.

Contact lens wearers need to be especially cautious. In

addition to all of the causes of eye inflammation listed here, contact lens use can cause dryness, abrasions, trapping of foreign bodies, or prolongation of infection.

If you wear contacts and the whites of your eyes become irritated or reddened for whatever reason, remove the contact lens from the affected eye and throw it away. Do not use a contact in that eye again until the eye is back to normal for at least 24 hours. If leaving the contact out for a day or two does not relieve your symptoms, see your family doctor or eye doctor. Sometimes what you think is merely an irritation may be a scratched cornea that requires medical attention.

46. Sinusitis

Picture this scenario. *You're* the doctor. Your patient has waited an hour to see you. He complains of congestion, headache, sinus pressure, and postnasal drainage. Yes, the drainage is yellow. No, he hasn't missed work. He winces when you tap his sinuses. He wants you to know how miserable he is. *You gotta do something, Doc.*

Is it sinusitis or is it a cold?

Sinusitis means inflammation of the lining of the sinus cavities. It does *not* always mean infection. From what I've seen in primary care medicine, doctors often—quite often—use the diagnosis "sinusitis" as an excuse to give antibiotics. It's what our patients want after all, at least most of them. Whether antibiotics work or not, patients *believe* in them.

But colds are much more common than sinus infections, and allergies can cause similar symptoms.

It's just a cold, you tell the patient. *No antibiotics are indicated.*

Your patient glares at you. *He* knows what he needs. The next day he calls your partner and demands an antibiotic—and gets it. No sense getting sued over amoxicillin.

Here's the point. Unless the situation is bad enough to make you feverish, or to make you miss work, or to make you look sick enough for an X-ray, it's probably just a cold—sinus irritation caused by a virus.

Here are seven tips to save money on sinusitis:

1. Ask your doctor if it's truly bacterial sinusitis. If he makes a convincing argument, then request a $4 antibiotic. Rarely do you need something more costly. The inexpensive antibiotics include amoxicillin, sulfa drugs, doxycycline, erythromycin, cephalexin, and ciprofloxacin. Of these, the first four are considered first-line antibiotics for respiratory infections.

2. Otherwise, what you want and need is symptom relief. We'll start with pain—facial pain, head pain, or even sometimes tooth pain. You'd be surprised how often a patient hasn't considered standard pain relievers such as Tylenol, aspirin, Advil, Motrin (ibuprofen), or Aleve—they all provide effective relief for most patients—for under $5.

3. Mucus. Snot. Phlegm. Take your pick. If you have excess mucus, you'll want to either dry it up or make it run thinner, like maple syrup in the spring (see #5 on this list).

Antihistamines such as Benadryl (diphenhydramine) and Zyrtec dry up mucus. This can be good or bad. For some people it provides real relief. For others, it makes them feel worse—they can't get the snot out (see #4 below). Over-the-counter medications are as good as prescription medications—most were prescription some time ago anyway—at a cost of under $10. Of the OTC antihistamines, the nonsedating drug Claritin (loratadine) works great for allergies, but Benadryl and Zyrtec often work better for symptoms associated with infection.

4. If you can't get the snot out, try nasal douching. When you have a clogged pipe, you run water through it. Same goes for the nose. Use a penny's worth of warm salt-water and run it through from one side to the other. This flushes out germs, mucus, chemicals, allergens (things you're allergic to), and sometimes foreign bodies. For a video from the Mayo clinic that shows you how to perform the irrigation, visit: www.mayoclinic.com/health/nasal-lavage/MM00552.

5. If you can't beat 'em, join 'em. Rather than dry up the mucus, many patients feel better if the mucus is allowed to flow more freely. Mucolytics—primarily guaifenesin, the active ingredient in Mucinex and many cough medicines—make mucus more watery. Then it feels like you're swallowing saliva rather than snot, just like you're supposed to. Don't spend $40 on a fancy product. Get a $7 store brand.

6. And next, my personal favorite: pseudoephedrine. In the good old days, a few years ago, you could buy pseu-

doephedrine over the counter. Now you have to ask a pharmacist for it, thanks to the meth labs. The new Sudafed PE contains phenylephrine, not nearly as effective in my experience. Pseudoephedrine opens the nasal/sinus passages, allowing mucus and air to flow more freely. It also has a bit of a drying effect. If I could choose only one therapy, this would be it—relief for under $10. Even though the medication is over the counter, prescription plans often cover it, often at a lower cost than buying it off the shelf. Common side effects include insomnia and palpitations, much like excess caffeine.

7. Ask your pharmacist for free advice. Tell your pharmacist your symptoms and she can tell you what medications will help you most. They deal with these medicines every day—skip the doctor and save 50 bucks. Since you're seeking symptom relief, be as specific as possible. If you have multiple symptoms, a multirelief medication may be your best bet.

47. Sprained ankle

A sprained ankle is rarely an emergency. So put your feet up and rest a spell.

By far the most common ankle sprain occurs as the foot rolls inward with the lateral ankle outward. This stretches and sometimes tears the ligament that connects the outer ankle bone to the foot. The outer part of the ankle, usually below the ankle bone, swells, hurts, and may bruise or feel unstable.

You should seek immediate medical attention if:

- The ankle is deformed, not just swollen
- A bone is sticking out
- You have poor circulation, diabetes, preexisting swelling, neuropathy, a skin infection, or other chronic problem

Otherwise it's safe to wait a bit—perhaps you won't need to see a doctor at all. While you're waiting, keep your ankle up and apply ice. Wrap it with an elastic bandage if it's continuing to swell. Take a couple Tylenol or ibuprofen and give the medicine at least an hour to work before deciding to see a doctor. You'll be waiting hours in the ER anyway. Give yourself a chance to recuperate at home.

Is the ankle stable? If you've already walked on the affected leg and didn't experience a feeling of instability it's probably not broken nor severely sprained. So far, so good. If you haven't tried walking, give it a whirl—carefully— making sure not to fall. If it seems unstable, stay off it and see your doctor. Unless it is obviously deformed, waiting until morning is fine.

Next, how's the pain? If it's not too bad it's probably not broken. However, you may need to seek medical attention if the pain isn't relieved with over-the-counter medications.

Also, if the ankle is quite swollen, feels unstable, but *doesn't* hurt as much as you'd expect it should, you may have ruptured the ligament completely, which will require casting or surgery or both. It is unlikely that casting or surgery will be done on an emergency basis. For otherwise healthy individuals (those without diabetes, chronic swelling, or poor circulation), this, too, can wait until morning.

For the typical patient with mild to moderate pain and swelling but with minimal instability, rest, ice, compression, and elevation (remember: RICE) are usually all it takes to heal a sprained ankle. If it hurts to walk, use crutches for a day or two. Crutches cost $20–$30 at your local drugstore without a prescription (or borrow them from a friend for greater savings). Get an ankle splint or gel cast, also available from your local pharmacy, for $10–$30 without a prescription, and wear it until your ankle seems fine. (Use it when you exercise for an extra week or two to prevent reinjury.) Apply an elastic wrap (an Ace wrap) to decrease swelling. Continue Tylenol or ibuprofen as needed, for a few days to a few weeks.

You should make steady progress, getting a little better each day. If not, see your doctor who will determine if you need an X-ray or further therapy. Second-degree sprains sometimes take months to heal, and occasionally require surgery.

48. Bee stings and bug bites

Yours truly is a perfect example of someone who seems allergic to bee stings and bug bites but isn't.

Mosquitoes love me and leave quarter-size welts that itch for hours. Deerfly bites swell to six inches across and last for days. Stings cause pain and swelling for a week, and chigger bites torture me for a month. All of these are local reactions.

Local reactions begin at the site of the bite or sting, usually causing an itchy, red, swollen spot that spreads outward in a symmetric pattern. Certain people develop larger local reactions than others, especially those with an allergic disposition, eczema, or asthma—like me.

You don't need to seek medical attention for a local reaction unless:

- You've been bitten by a poisonous critter (know the ones in your area)
- You're having trouble breathing (call 911)
- The bite or sting appears infected (look for pus, increasing redness, pain, or fever)
- You've suffered such a large number of stings or bites that you're in danger of a generalized reaction (call 911) (probably at least five or more stings)
- What you think may be a spider bite is actually a methicillin-resistant staph aureus (MRSA) infection that requires antibiotics. Unless you've seen what bit you, don't assume you have a spider bite.

Save money on local reactions by:

- Avoiding biting/stinging insects
- Using insect repellant
- Treating yourself at home using antihistamines and hydrocortisone cream (see #31 and #97 for more information)

For a beautiful slide show of bugs and the rashes they may cause, visit WebMD at: www.webmd.com/allergies/slide show-bad-bugs.

An allergic reaction, on the other hand, produces symptoms somewhere other than the site of the bite or sting. *Seek medical attention* if you can't breathe normally or if you develop hives, wheezing, palpitations, nausea, headache, fainting, or other strange symptoms—call 911 if needed. *Such a reaction can be life-threatening.*

For a true allergy, your doctor will likely prescribe an EpiPen for future use. Make sure you know how to use it before leaving the pharmacy—and keep it on hand when you're outside.

For local reactions over-the-counter antihistamines (see #97) will lessen the itch and may decrease the redness. Apply ice to a sting to help the pain or use over-the-counter pain relievers. Hydrocortisone cream also soothes the itch. Bacitracin helps a bite that appears mildly infected.

Atopic (reactive) people like me may also be extremely sensitive to insect sprays, making their use a challenge. Last year I experimented with the Off! PowerPad Lamp, a small lantern-type device that uses a candle to warm a chemical-impregnated pad. I was totally delighted with its effectiveness. If you'll be sitting in one place outdoors, I highly recommend giving it a try. The Off! Clip-On is intended to provide protection as you work outside, but the insect-repellant effect may not keep up with your movement.

49. Stomach flu (acute gastroenteritis)

Save your money and stay home. You rarely need a doctor for a simple case of the stomach flu.

The biggest reason patients require medical intervention for stomach flu is dehydration.

Of course, it's important to have the right diagnosis. If all your coworkers and two of your children have the stomach flu, you probably do, too. On the other hand, many other conditions can masquerade as stomach flu including food poisoning, urinary tract infections, gallbladder inflammation, ulcers, pregnancy, and stomach irritation from a variety of medications.

But assuming you have a typical virus that causes nausea, vomiting, fatigue, and maybe diarrhea or fever, stay hydrated and stay at home.

There's no medication to cure the condition anyway. However, medication may lessen your symptoms. Meclizine (see #93) can help the nausea and vomiting. Loperamide (see #94) can reduce the diarrhea. If heartburn or stomach irritability occurs, the H_2s or PPIs may be useful (see #91–#92). Avoid stomach irritants (see #92) and NSAID medications such as aspirin and ibuprofen (see #96). Alka-Seltzer is a curious concoction, containing both aspirin (bad for the stomach) and an antacid (good for the stomach). It should probably be avoided during a bout of stomach flu. Avoid alcohol use as well.

Remaining well hydrated is the goal of therapy. And that doesn't just mean water. In fact, plain water isn't absorbed as well as sugary saltwater. (IV fluid is sugary saltwater, too.) The salt is needed to replace salt lost in the stool, and sugar is needed to increase the absorption of salt and water.

Gatorade and other sports drinks are appropriate oral re-hydration therapy in otherwise healthy adults and children. Buy the regular kind, not the low-calorie variety when you're sick. Artificial sweeteners don't improve the absorption of fluids like sugar does, and since you're not likely to be eating much, the extra calories may perk you up. (For care of infants, the elderly, and patients with chronic illnesses such as diabetes or heart failure, consult your physician.)

Sports drinks are balanced solutions of sugar and electrolytes (salts). It's possible to make your own. The Rehydration Project gives the following recipe for oral rehydration solution at www.rehydrate.org/solutions/homemade.htm:

- One level teaspoon of salt
- Eight level teaspoons of sugar
- One liter (5 cups) of clean water
- Optional: add ½ cup fruit juice, such as apple juice

Start using the replacement solution as soon as the illness begins, and continue until you can eat and drink normal foods again. See your doctor if you're not better within a few days.

50. Yeast infections (monilia, candidiasis)

Anyone who's ever baked bread knows yeast needs a warm, moist environment to propagate. The same is true of yeast infections of the body.

Warm, moist areas of the body prone to yeast infections include:

- Groin
- Diaper area and around the rectum
- Vagina and surrounding areas
- Skin folds such as under the abdomen, armpit, or breast
- Tongue and mouth

Itching, discharge, and redness are the hallmarks of vaginal yeast infections. Beware these same symptoms may be caused by certain STDs and occasionally by urine infections.

Infected skin exhibits red patches or bumps, or itching, especially in the diaper area. Skin folds under the armpit, breast, or abdomen may also exhibit an odor or slight wetness.

Yeast infections of the mouth (thrush) usually cause white spots on the tongue or the inside of the cheeks, along with some redness and soreness.

Although yeast infections may occur for no apparent reason, recent antibiotic use and diabetes are common triggers.

Steroid pills, injections, or inhalers also make yeast infections more likely.

The cost of treating yeast infections has decreased dramatically in recent years, and treatments for under $10 are available for every site of infection.

Yeast infections of the skin are treated about the same as fungal infections—see #99 for detailed information. Keeping skin folds dry can minimize the risk of yeast intertrigo (yeast infection of moist skin folds).

Vaginal yeast infections are also preventable to a degree. Avoid unnecessary antibiotics and diabetics, and keep your blood sugar under control. Some people swear that probiotics and yogurt (live culture) make a difference. The thinking is that replenishing normal bacteria prevents harmful bacteria and yeast from growing.

If you're certain you have a vaginal yeast infection, use one of the OTC preparations and save the cost of an office visit. Gyne-Lotrimin, Monistat, and Vagistat (or generics of these) were once prescription medications that are now available OTC for $10 to $20. They come in various regimens, from one to seven days, and a variety of creams and suppositories. (See appendix 2 for Web sites.) One word of caution—if you are continuing to take an antibiotic or steroid you may need to extend or repeat the anti-yeast treatment.

The most popular *prescription* drug for yeast infections is the 150-milligram single-dose Diflucan oral tablet, which costs $15 to $30 per pill. It is now available as generic fluconazole on most $4 lists (one for $4, three for $10). Some pharmacies offer the 100-milligram tablet at a greater discount, for example, 10 tablets for $4. Ask your doctor to prescribe multiple pills if you are prone to recurrent infections.

The vaginal yeast creams may also be used for yeast diaper rash. Of course, it's better to prevent the problem in the first place. Keep your baby dry. Prolonged contact with urine or feces can cause a chemical irritation or burn. (Adults can get a "diaper rash" for the same reasons.) Some children are more susceptible to these chemical irritants—use a *thick* layer of Desitin (zinc oxide) as a barrier cream. A regular diaper rash may become infected with yeast, creating a dual problem. Also, if your baby has taken an antibiotic and *isn't* prone to recurrent diaper rashes, a yeast diaper rash is extremely likely. Yeast diaper rash can be treated with OTC Lotrimin or other antifungal or anti-yeast cream for about $5. Only if the rash persists is a trip to the doctor necessary.

Prescription nystatin oral suspension for *thrush* (in the mouth) is priced at $4 at many pharmacies (see #16). If you find a higher price at your drugstore, ask about price matching (see #13). Mycelex Troche is another common prescription, but costs over $100 (generic about $70). If your doctor prescribes this medication and cost (including higher co-pay) is a concern, request the generic nystatin.

As for prevention of thrush, once again, avoid antibiotics whenever possible. Close attention to blood sugar control is essential in diabetics. Denture-wearers do well to remove their teeth daily for cleaning. Brush your mouth thoroughly while they're out. If you have asthma or COPD and use a steroid inhaler, be sure to rinse your mouth afterward or take a drink of water to rinse the steroid away.

Eating yeast-leavened bread will not give you a yeast infection—the yeast has been killed with baking. We all have yeast in our colon, anyway, but normally our own immunity holds it at bay. Only when our body's defense mechanisms are lowered or altered can a yeast infection take hold.

CHAPTER SIX

Save Money on Medical Testing

51. Can that X-ray wait?

People with insurance worry about the cost of their insurance, not about the cost of medical care.

People without insurance worry about the cost of all medical care, especially medical testing.

An ankle X-ray may cost a few hundred dollars, an ultrasound about $1,000, a CAT scan $1,500–$2,000, and an MRI perhaps twice that. Not small ticket items.

The decision to order an X-ray is not nearly as black and white as you may think. There are many shades of gray, depending on severity of symptoms, availability of X-ray equipment, and the element of clinical judgment.

Patient reliability is an additional factor, one within your control. In an ER where the doctor doesn't know you personally, you're much more likely to receive extensive testing than if you visit your personal physician, who hopefully knows you well. If your doctor trusts you to follow through with a mutually agreed-upon treatment plan, and to call if you experience additional problems, he's much less likely to order

X-rays at the outset. Many problems resolve over the course of a day or a week. It's extremely helpful to have a doctor who knows your normal state of health and appearance. An emergency room doctor lacks this benefit and cannot judge from experience whether you are a reliable person (see #2).

A doctor will be more willing to rely on his or her personal clinical judgment (as opposed to X-rays) if he or she has confidence in you. *Will you follow directions? Will you return if the problem worsens? Is the cost savings worth the degree of uncertainty?*

Examples of problems where the possibility of deferring an X-ray is a consideration include:

- Sprained ankles, feet, and wrists
- Potentially fractured toes
- Painful knees
- Low-back pain
- Cough or wheezing
- Headaches
- Stomach problems
- Possible kidney stones

An experienced doctor's opinion is worth more than an X-ray—and costs less as well. Ask your doctor if an X-ray is mandatory, or if it could be deferred a few days or weeks, perhaps allowing your body to heal in the meantime. Ask what to watch for that would make an X-ray advisable. Be compliant with whatever treatment your doctor prescribes. Develop a contingency plan for potentially serious outcomes.

Work toward developing a trusting relationship with your doctor and you may save hundreds to thousands of dollars.

52. Ask for an "HMO discount"

It's hardly fair, but the fact is that self-pay patients pay the most for medical testing.

At Walmart everybody pays the same price. Not so with medical testing—it's more like a fresh-air market where the best haggler gets the best deal.

Health maintenance organizations (HMOs), preferred provider organizations (PPOs), Medicare, Medicaid, and other insurance plans receive substantial discounts on medical testing including blood work, X-rays, MRIs, and nearly everything else.

Negotiated discounts with the "big players" whittle the profit margin on medical testing down considerably, with reimbursement rates sometimes less than the cost of performing the test. The self-pay patient may unwittingly help subsidize the discounts insured patients receive.

No discounts are offered to self-pay patients—at least not unless you ask. (Of course, if everyone receives unsustainable discounts, medical providers will simply go out of business—but that's not our concern at the moment.)

As a self-pay patient, you can safely assume that whatever price you've been billed is the highest price for a given test. You can also safely assume that someone else is paying less.

For example, a urinalysis that you may be charged $40 for could easily be discounted down to only $3 or $4 by insurance companies (an unsustainable discount, I might add). Doctors commonly charge about $18 for a venipuncture (a blood draw), but Medicare pays only $3, the rest of which is written off. An EKG billed at $60 could be discounted down to as little as a third as much by a contracted health insurance plan.

It certainly doesn't seem fair—especially to the self-pay patient.

So, when you receive a bill (or even better, before undergoing medical testing), go to the billing office at the appropriate facility, explain your situation, and ask for what I call the "HMO discount," the amount that an HMO would pay for the same service you received. Tell them that you don't have health insurance. Ask if they have a sliding fee scale for uninsured patients. If they don't, ask if they know of a local facility that does. Ask if paying up front entitles you to a reduction in your bill. Merely being uninsured *may* be sufficient to trigger a discount; however, it is possible the hospital or facility will require financial means testing (see #54). The billing office may or may not be willing to adjust their fees, but you can be sure they won't if you don't ask. (See also chapter 7, "Save Money on Hospital Expenses.")

Whereas hospitals and large health care facilities absorb these discounts into their overall budget, if you ask your private doctor for a discount on tests performed in his office, this money will come directly from his pocket. Don't forget to say thank-you (see #10).

53. Comparison shop for blood work

Just as a designer dress may cost twice as much at a designer store, so blood work may cost considerably more at one facility versus another. A soft drink you buy for a quarter at the grocery store may cost ten times that at a movie theater. Likewise, the "retail" markup on blood work is priced according to what the market will bear.

Perhaps it seems unethical for this to occur in the field of health care, but it is a business, and a profit must be generated.

One difference between health care costs and other retail pricing is that health care charges are "invisible," neither advertised nor displayed. However, it is still possible to comparison shop.

To begin, you need an order from your doctor for the required laboratory testing. It would be helpful if the order is legible, so you know what to ask for.

There are three common options for lab testing: your doctor's office, a hospital outpatient lab, and independent medical labs. Most hospitals maintain their own laboratories for frequently performed tests but send blood to regional reference labs for uncommon tests. Your doctor may perform blood tests in her own facility or draw blood to send to a local independent lab or to a reference lab. Independent medical labs and some hospitals have conveniently located "drawing stations" (small offices where blood is drawn but not tested on site). Search the yellow pages or online for medical and/or clinical labs (laboratories) in your area.

With order in hand, ask the price of the ordered tests, and whether there are any hidden fees such as additional venipuncture charges, transportation charges, or physician interpretation of results. At a private medical office, the receptionist or nurse can give you this information. At a hospital or independent lab, ask for the billing department. You can also check online for prices at your local hospital, though not all hospital Web sites list this information.

It is useful to know some of the abbreviations doctors use when ordering tests:

- BMP = basic metabolic profile
- CBC = complete blood count
- CMP = complete metabolic profile
- C & S = culture & sensitivity
- FBS = fasting blood sugar
- H & H = hemoglobin & hematocrit
- HgA1C = hemoglobin A1C (average blood sugar)
- Lipids = cholesterol profile
- RBS = random blood sugar
- TSH = thyroid stimulating hormone
- T3 or T4 = thyroid hormone level
- UA = urinalysis

Check at least three lab providers, and make a chart for comparison. It doesn't hurt to ask if a self-pay discount is available. Although hospitals and other large facilities often charge more, they are also more likely to offer an income-based sliding fee schedule. On the other hand, your personal physician knows you better and may be more motivated to help you.

If you have insurance, check which lab is covered before having your blood drawn, or you may be in for a costly surprise. Insurance companies negotiate for discounted pricing, contracting with labs that offer the best deal. Don't assume testing is covered at every local facility. Private physicians usually contract with only one or two labs, which may or may not be the same labs that your insurance has contracted with. Some physicians have discontinued office-based testing and blood-drawing altogether due to decreasing insurance payments and the increasing hassle factor. If a doctor will get paid only $3 for a venipuncture procedure that costs $10 to $15 to perform, it makes little business sense to offer the service.

54. Financial means testing

If you're facing a costly hospitalization (or expensive outpatient testing or treatment) and have a choice of facility, consider choosing a nonprofit hospital, a charity hospital, a teaching hospital, or public hospital.

Public hospitals are "safety net" hospitals that care for all patients, regardless of ability to pay. (Of course, patients with the ability to pay are expected to pay.) To locate a public hospital in your area, visit the National Association of Public Hospitals and Health Systems at: www.naph.org or call 202-585-0100.

Hospitals sponsored by religious organizations (hospitals with the words saint, Catholic, Lutheran, mercy, Baptist,

Presbyterian, charity, etc. in their name) are also dedicated to helping the uninsured and offer income-based discounts.

Teaching hospitals (hospitals associated with a medical school) employ resident physicians (physicians in training) who work with the oversight of fully trained doctors. Teaching hospitals care for the nation's poor and uninsured as well. To locate a teaching hospital in your state, visit the Association of American Medical Colleges Web site at www.aamc.org. If you do not have access to a computer, go to your local public library and ask a librarian to help you find this information.

For-profit hospitals are investor-owned. Like any for-profit business, they try to garner a profit for their shareholders. They may be less likely to offer discounts than nonprofit hospitals.

Many nonprofit hospitals receive subsidies to allow them to provide reduced cost care or even free care to lower income families or individuals. It's not surprising that this is not well publicized—hospitals are not looking to go out of business.

Save money by talking to the billing department or a social worker ahead of time (or as soon as possible after hospital admission) to learn if the hospital offers a sliding fee scale or discounted fees according to patient or family income.

Of course, hospitals will not simply take your word for it that you cannot afford to pay. They will require *financial means testing* (or analysis) to determine if you're eligible.

This means that you will need to provide proof of your income, assets, and liabilities. The hospital will want to know the same information a bank would require to process a mortgage loan.

Start a file to include the following information:

- A copy of your social security card
- A copy of your driver's license
- A copy of your birth certificate and that of your spouse and/or children
- Three most recent pay stubs for you, your spouse, and any other household member
- Tax returns for the past three years
- Proof of child support, paid or received
- Proof of alimony, paid or received
- Proof of residence (tax or utility bill)
- Proof of marital status
- Proof of student status
- Proof of citizenship or alien status
- Recurring bills including mortgage payment, car payment, and credit card bills
- Monthly rent, utility and phone bills
- Proof of assets including home ownership, vehicles, stocks, bonds, and bank accounts

Though it may take a few hours to organize this information, it could save thousands of dollars in the long run. A hospital may not require every document listed above or might ask for a few others, but having this information readily available should speed up the process. Since the hospital won't benefit from giving you a discount, the onus is on you to keep track of the process. Keep copies of everything, make a log of all communications, call back if you haven't received an answer, and, most importantly, *don't give up.*

55. Health department services

Local county or city health departments are funded by your tax dollars. They offer free or reduced cost services, many of which are targeted at populations likely to have difficulty affording medical care, including students, uninsured adults, pregnant women, infants, and children. They also offer services for the population at large, including vaccines, TB tests, and travel immunization advice.

To locate your local health department, check the government section of your phone book, or search online, or call your local hospital or medical society for information. The Health Guide USA provides an online listing of over 1,200 health departments by state and county at www .healthguideusa.org.

Local health department services may vary, depending on the needs of the community. Commonly they include:

- AIDS/HIV testing
- Alcohol and drug abuse programs
- Animal bite and rabies information
- Blood lead level testing
- Breast cancer screening, including mammograms
- Carbon monoxide testing
- Cervical cancer screening, including Pap smears

- Child health services and vaccines
- Diabetes screening and treatment
- Employment physicals
- Family planning services, including contraceptives
- Flu shots and pneumonia shots
- High cholesterol screening and treatment
- Hypertension screening and treatment
- Prenatal clinic for pregnant women
- Prostate cancer screening including PSA tests
- Quit smoking classes
- Refugee program
- Sexually transmitted disease clinic including HIV/AIDS
- Travel immunizations and advice
- Tuberculosis testing and/or treatment
- Women Infants and Children (WIC) Program
- Women's health clinic

The circumstances under which a person might receive discounted services from a local health department are many and varied.

For example, a young woman with limited financial means could schedule a female exam at her health department women's health clinic for free or at reduced cost. In addition to a Pap smear, she may receive counseling and/or treatment regarding family planning and sexually transmitted diseases. If it turns out she's pregnant, she can be referred to the prenatal clinic and WIC clinic for additional services.

Uninsured families may have a private physician, yet be unable to afford the multiple checkups and vaccines young children require. Health departments offer well-child exams and "baby shots" for free or at greatly reduced cost, as well as state-mandated screening for lead exposure and anemia.

College students away from home or young adults out on their own can visit the local health department for free or discounted flu shots, alcohol and drug abuse programs, and STD testing and treatment.

Workers who require a physical or TB test as a condition for employment can receive the needed screening for a minimal fee (or free). Anyone can receive a tetanus update or advice on immunizations required for overseas travel. Blood testing is often available at discounted rates for middle-aged patients at increased risk for diabetes, high blood pressure, or high cholesterol.

Call your local health department and ask about your medical needs. If the health department doesn't have the means to serve you, it should be able to refer you to a provider who can.

56. An appointment for test results?

I've often heard patients complain that their doctor made them come back just to tell them their tests were normal. *Why did I have to wait two hours when he could have told me over the phone?* they wonder.

Good point. Your time is valuable, too.

A follow-up appointment to review results of medical tests should have a specific goal, not merely the conveyance of a negative result.

There is no set standard for requiring a patient to return

to the office to receive test results. Some offices work on the "if you don't hear from us, don't worry" plan. I never liked that plan—what if the results were lost in the mail or your phone was disconnected? Other physicians require every patient to return to their office for test results. While this does increase business and allows more time for questions, it's often unnecessary and costs the patient time and money.

At my own office, my medical assistant calls every patient with every test result and a plan for what to do next. As a rule, the next step has already been discussed before the test is ordered. If the test shows problem X, then we'll proceed with treatment Y. If the tests are all normal, then no follow-up may be needed. However, if the results are quite involved I usually do request a follow-up appointment for a detailed discussion.

You can often save the cost of a follow-up appointment by discussing your options ahead of time. Whenever your doctor orders a test, ask what the next step will be. If the test is normal, do you need to return? Do you need an additional test? Do you need to be reevaluated at some point? If the test shows a problem, do you need medication? A referral to a specialist? A follow-up visit? This discussion may extend your initial office visit a few minutes (see #5 and #6), but one longer visit costs less than two separate appointments. If you do need a follow-up appointment for an acute problem, perhaps you can combine it with a visit for a chronic problem such as diabetes or hypertension.

Another option is a telephone appointment. Traditionally, doctors have only been paid for time spent face to face with a patient, making them understandably reluctant to spend much time on the phone. However, in this era of instant communication, this practice is changing.

Ask your doctor if a telephone appointment for test results would be appropriate. Some insurance companies are beginning to reimburse for phone appointments. If your doctor does not offer phone appointments, that doesn't necessarily mean he'd refuse if you offer to pay for his time. Generally charges for phone appointments are somewhat less than for office visits, especially if they are short and to the point. But if your doctor has a contract with an insurance company that *doesn't* pay for phone appointments and if that contract won't allow him to bill extra for the service, it's not likely your doctor will agree to a phone appointment. You wouldn't want to extend your day either for work you don't get paid for, would you?

Another consideration is whether you'd want to hear bad news on the phone. Most doctors are reluctant to deliver news of cancer or terminal illness via such an impersonal means.

If your doctor requests that you return for test results, organize your thoughts and be prepared with questions. Don't leave the office wondering why you came. Make sure you understand what your plan of care is, what you can do to help yourself, what additional problems you might encounter, and when you should return and why. Make notes and bring a relative along to help with questions if needed. Ask for a copy of test results for your personal health file. Ask enough questions to understand your condition, but stick to the point. Your doctor will appreciate your organization and focus.

57. Take advantage of health fair screenings

Health care providers show up at many community events to man booths offering free medical tests. Examples of organizations that participate in health fairs from time to time include:

- Hospitals
- Health departments
- Local physicians
- Home medical service providers
- Community health clinics
- Visiting nurse associations
- Pharmacies
- Hearing aid suppliers
- Medical schools
- Extended care facilities
- Local medical societies

The so-called health fair may be part of an actual fair or an event organized at a church, school, shopping area, hospital, or community center. These venues are intended to raise public awareness and are viewed as a form of advertising.

But they're also an opportunity for you to obtain free (or

inexpensive) health care. Usually you are given a written copy of your test results, which you can give to your doctor and discuss at your next appointment.

Check your local newspaper and listen for radio or television announcements. You might also want to call your local hospital community outreach office, health department, or medical association and ask if they offer periodic testing on-site at a reduced fee.

The following are examples of services offered at community-sponsored health fairs:

- Anemia (CBC) screening
- Blood chemistry tests
- Carotid artery screening (but read #30)
- Cholesterol screening
- Circulation screening
- Dental screening
- Fasting blood sugar screening
- Hearing tests
- Hypertension (blood pressure) screening
- Mammograms
- Osteoporosis screening
- PSA (prostate) testing (but read #27)
- Vision screening

Enjoy the fair and all the health food you can find there, but better get your blood work checked before you hit the concession stand.

58. Lengthen the interval between tests

Like much of life, medical care is organized according to the phases of the moon, the seasons, and the revolution of the earth around the sun.

In other words, intervals for periodic testing and follow-up are determined in weeks, months, and years. Pharmacies give refills by the month or the quarter. The annual physical is done annually.

But there's nothing magic—only convenient—about the standard interval of testing.

Anyone who has lab tests on a regular basis is a candidate for savings based on extending the interval between these tests. For patients who have monthly blood work, say for a blood thinner or lithium level, if your results have been fairly stable your physician might be willing to extend the interval from four to five weeks, saving two blood draws and two sets of labs a year, easily $100 or more.

For diabetics receiving blood tests every three months, your doctor may be willing to extend the interval to four (or perhaps six) months *if* you do your part to keep your blood sugar regulated. Your doctor will not extend this interval if you do not take your medicines regularly or if your sugar is not controlled, or if you have other complications.

For patients receiving annual blood work, say for high cholesterol or hypothyroidism, if your levels are stable and you're compliant with your medicine, your doctor may be willing to do blood work every 15 to 18 months, saving you the cost of one set of labs every three years, again easily hundreds of dollars.

In a person without significant risk factors, other tests might be spread *a little* further apart as well—EKGs, mammograms, Pap smears, colonoscopies.

Medical research does not test for every possible screening interval. Convenient intervals are chosen to coincide with daily life. For example, a Pap smear or mammogram every 15 or 18 months might be every bit as good as testing every 12 months, but people generally don't plan their lives in intervals of 15 or 18 months. Still, a responsible adult looking to save money could keep a calendar of medical testing and discuss this option with her doctor.

The greater risk of extending an interval from a year, say, to a year and a half is that perhaps the test will be ignored or forgotten altogether. Partnering with your doctor is essential (see #2) to determine what is in your best interest.

59. Making sense of strep and mono tests

A sore throat is one of the most common illnesses where lab testing adds significantly to the expense of an office visit. A strep throat test is frequently ordered when a patient presents with a sore throat, often before the patient is seen by the physician. Mononucleosis testing is sometimes added when a strep test is negative, especially when the patient is a teenager or young adult.

Strep testing begins with a rapid strep test that detects Group A streptococcal bacteria in the throat. It takes only about five minutes to perform the test. If the result is positive, your doctor will diagnose you or your child with strep throat, although the rare patient may have a false-positive result. False-negative tests are somewhat more common, occurring in perhaps 2–5 percent of negative rapid strep tests. Your doctor may order a strep culture to confirm you don't have strep. The strep culture is considered a bit more accurate but takes at least a day or two for results to become available. A third type of strep test is rarely ordered (an antistreptolysin O titer) and takes weeks to be detectable in the blood.

Mono testing generally consists of a complete blood count ($50 to $80) and/or an antibody test ($20 to $50). Infectious mononucleosis often does not show up on blood tests until the patient has been ill a good week or more. There are actually two types of mono (named for a preponderance of mononuclear cells in the blood): Epstein-Barr virus and cytomegalovirus. Cytomegalovirus does not show up on a standard mono test.

People with good insurance don't ask about the cost of testing. Patients without insurance do ask—and with good reason. For a self-pay patient, the cost of strep testing adds considerably to a visit with your doctor, at least $25 more, and possibly two to four times that.

Before we get to the finer points of strep testing, please read #43, *Laryngitis and pharyngitis (sore throat)*.

Here are several issues to discuss with your doctor to help you keep your costs down:

First, *is a strep test going to make a difference in treatment?* If your doctor plans to give you an antibiotic regardless of the test result, there's very little reason to perform the test.

Second, *what is the plan if the initial rapid strep test is neg-*

ative? Some doctors will conclude you don't have strep. However, since there is still a slight chance you do have strep despite the negative test, other doctors may order a confirmatory strep culture. When cost is a concern, you might want to skip the rapid test and wait a day or two for the culture results. There's no harm in waiting.

Of course, in our *now* culture, we want results *now*. But, if you have strep, starting an antibiotic a day or two later makes practically no difference in how quickly you recover. The likelihood of developing rheumatic fever is no greater waiting even up to a week after symptoms begin before beginning a course of antibiotics.

Third, *issues of contagion should be considered.* If you have a dozen children and six have sore throats, testing one or two of them may help you decide what to do about the rest.

Also, strep throat is not contagious after 24 hours of antibiotic therapy (perhaps a little longer if fever persists). If you'll have to stay home to care for yourself or your children, testing for strep may help minimize your time off work, saving you money in the form of wages not lost.

Fourth, though the charge for one or both strep tests may run $25–$100, reimbursement from insurance companies is *far* less than that. If you are self-pay, remind your doctor you have no insurance. Ask whether you really need a test, ask how much time off work you'll require, ask if your doctor will treat other family members without an appointment if you have a positive test and other family members come down with similar symptoms. If testing is in your best interest, ask if your doctor would consider a discount on strep testing.

Fifth, testing for mononucleosis is a consideration in a teenager or young adult with a negative strep test. However, unless your teen is extremely ill, waiting a week or so to test is reasonable for two reasons: 1) the test is often negative in the first week, meaning a negative result does not assure your child doesn't have mono; and 2) mono often resolves within a week or two anyway.

Since there is no cure for mono, what's the purpose of the test? I generally order mono testing only in a person who has a prolonged sore throat and is sick enough to miss work or school beyond several days, and therefore needs an answer to explain his prolonged absence. Rarely, I order the test to make sure my patient doesn't have a more serious illness.

If you are concerned about the cost of mono testing, keep the above in mind. And if you're uninsured, don't be afraid to ask for a discount.

60. Who reads your X-ray?

Medical bills can be confusing even to the medical professional. For the patient it can be a nightmare.

How can a doctor charge you when he's never even seen you? One answer has to do with interpretation of medical tests. EKGs and X-rays are two common examples. Lung function tests (spirometry) and biopsy results may generate additional reading fees as well.

Most hospitals and other large health care providers have a system in place whereby every EKG is interpreted by a cardiologist and every X-ray is read by a radiologist. These specialists have a right to charge for the work they perform, even though they've never seen you in person.

However, smaller facilities do not necessarily require that every test be reviewed by a specialist. A family physician or internist may perform a test in his or her own office and interpret the result personally, with the option of sending the test on to a specialist at a later time. Sending the test out incurs an additional charge.

Quite often a primary care physician will perform a test and need to act on the result immediately without benefit of an outside opinion. And quite often the interpretation is straightforward—especially if the test shows an easily apparent problem.

If an EKG shows you're having a heart attack, your doctor will send you to the ER—there's no need to get a second interpretation days later. If your X-ray shows your leg is broken, you'll need a cast—not another bill.

I expect that specialists who interpret these tests would disagree with me. It's true they have more expertise in their particular field. It's also true that when a patient is seen in an acute setting by a primary care doctor, the physician has to make a decision based on the information at hand. If the additional, delayed interpretation will not impact treatment, it probably isn't necessary.

If you're paying your own way and your doctor performs a test in his or her own office, ask whether you'll be receiving bills from any outside doctors, and whether it's truly necessary to obtain these outside opinions. Ask your doctor how confident she is of her own interpretation and whether a second opinion is truly necessary. Doctors in large facilities probably have no say in the matter, whereas physicians in small, private offices do.

You could easily save $20 to $50—or more—if your doctor relies on her own judgment. *But listen to your doctor*—if your physician insists on an outside reading, she's only doing it in your best interest.

CHAPTER SEVEN

Save Money on Hospital Expenses

61. Don't go—unless you have to

The hospital is the most expensive place to obtain health care. One trip to the ER will likely cost over $1,000, and a few days as an inpatient at least 10 grand.

Uninsured (and underinsured) patients are understandably distressed at the thought of spending their life savings on medical care. Sometimes, though, you can save money by avoiding the hospital. (Also see #1, 2, 3, and 8.)

First, *don't put off going if it's a true emergency*—like a suspected heart attack, or stroke, or dangerous bleeding. *Call 911*.

If it's not an emergency, call your doctor first. If your doctor thinks you should be hospitalized, ask about other options.

The need for hospitalization is not always a black-and-white issue. Severity, type, and course of illness are all major determining factors. Other coexisting diseases a patient may have play into the decision as well. For example, a patient with pneumonia *and* diabetes is more likely to be hospitalized than a patient with pneumonia alone.

But there is an important additional factor that is within your control: your reliability and trustworthiness as a patient. If your doctor knows and trusts you, your physician will be much more willing to consider treating a serious illness as an outpatient. If, on the other hand, your doctor has reason to doubt you, he will err on the side of hospital admission.

In the doctor-patient relationship, trustworthiness on the part of the patient is built by keeping your appointments, knowing your medicines and taking them as prescribed, reporting symptoms accurately, taking an active interest in your health care, remembering what was discussed in previous visits, demonstrating common sense, and following through on ordered tests or therapy.

Patients who don't demonstrate these traits, especially those who are found to lie repeatedly, build a reputation for unreliability. If your physician cannot trust you to comply with an outpatient treatment program, he is much more likely to recommend hospitalization where someone else can keep an eye on you.

Of course, some people have difficulty with the above recommendations due to memory problems, language barriers, poor hearing, or low IQ. They, too, are more likely to be hospitalized unless they have a caregiver whom the doctor trusts.

For a serious illness, what option is there other than hospitalization? Daily (or even twice daily) office visits are an alternative for certain patients. Seeing your doctor in the office five days in a row is less expensive than a single day in the hospital. Your physician must feel confident that you will follow his or her instructions and that you will take your medication as prescribed.

Sometimes doctors administer IV fluids, breathing treatments, or antibiotic injections in the office, all much less costly than receiving the same treatment in a hospital. Blood tests and X-rays can be obtained as an outpatient and repeated in a few days if necessary. The following illnesses, *when not severe*, are examples of problems that might be considered for close outpatient follow-up in place of hospitalization *in a reliable patient*:

- Pneumonia or COPD
- Urinary tract infection
- Vomiting and dehydration
- Uncontrolled diabetes
- Skin and soft-tissue infections
- Congestive heart failure

What sort of patient are you? For most of us, the decision is within our control. Being a reliable patient may save you thousands of dollars on hospital care.

62. Bring your own medications

Don't pay $5 for an aspirin if you can bring your own. There's no standard for what hospitals charge patients for an aspirin, but you can be sure it's a lot more than what you'd pay at your local pharmacy.

If you're going to be hospitalized and need to keep costs down, ask about bringing your own medicines along with you, and ask about administering them yourself. This includes daily medications for high blood pressure, cholesterol, diabetes, arthritis, asthma, COPD, allergies, GERD, seizures, back pain, depression, birth control, heart disease, glaucoma, or any other chronic condition. Types of medicines to consider bringing include pills, patches, inhalers, injections, eye drops, nose sprays, and creams.

The worst they can do is say no. Some hospitals are worried about liability issues. Others have a common sense approach— you were taking the same medications at home anyway, so why not in the hospital? It also depends on your reason for admission and what additional meds you'll need. Certain medications are commonly discontinued during hospitalization, for example, oral diabetic medication, due to the risk of low blood sugars in patients who are eating poorly.

But if you are going to be taking the same medications in the hospital that you were taking at home, bring two or three days worth of medicine *in the original prescription bottles* to the hospital. (Someone can replenish them later if needed, and in case of accidental loss, you don't want to lose a whole month's supply.) If you're diabetic, bring your blood glucose monitor and blood sugar log with you, as well as insulin and insulin needles. If the hospital won't allow you to use them, you can always send them back home.

Bringing an up-to-date medication list to the hospital is an excellent idea. The nurses will bless you for it. Include medication name, dose, frequency of dosing, prescribing doctor's name, and reason for taking. List drug allergies and intolerances as well.

Most hospitals don't keep every medication on hand. They work from a formulary, which includes one or two cost-effective options from each therapeutic class, medications that may or may not be the same as those your doctor has prescribed. If they substitute a different medication while you're in the hospital, you need to ask if you should take your previous medications when you return home.

If you're not permitted to use your own medications, when you're discharged, at least make sure you take any leftovers from the hospital home with you, including inhalers, creams, or opened containers. Don't forget any disposables such as plastic bed pans, incentive spirometers, emesis basins, and anything else the hospital is going to discard anyway—you've already been charged for them. Ask for the oxygen tubing if you like—it'll be in the trash soon otherwise.

If you take your own medicines, check your bill when you receive it to make sure you weren't charged for your own pills. However, if a nurse had to observe and document every time you took your medication, there may be a nursing charge for medication administration. If the charge seems out of line, don't hesitate to ask whether a discount is appropriate.

63. Request an itemized bill

Hospital bills are like cell phone bills. Normally, your carrier sends you only a summary of minutes used and corresponding charges. But if you ask, or go online, you can get details of every single call to each and every person.

The same is true of hospital bills. I've received such a bill myself—$10,000 for a day and a half in the hospital. No explanation of what that covered. Just pay the balance, thank you very much.

Like most people, since insurance covered the bulk of the charges, I didn't question it. But you'd better believe I'd look closer if I were footing the bill.

An itemized hospital bill should list every charge incurred during a hospital visit, excluding physician charges (see #67–#68). Every pill, every dressing, every X-ray, daily room charges—everything. And like checking out at your favorite mega-mart, mistakes do happen: tests are ordered, then cancelled; different personnel may input duplicate charges; meds are ordered, and then changed. Many opportunities for billing errors exist.

Go over your itemized bill with a fine-tooth comb. If two chest X-rays are listed but you remember only one, ask to see proof. If pharmacy charges are listed for medications you brought from home, discuss it with a patient account representative. If you were charged for five days of oxygen but used it only once, go ahead and challenge what may be a discrepancy. You probably won't recognize every charge, so ask—it's reasonable to know what you're paying for.

It's tough thinking about hospital bills when you don't feel well. If you find the process too difficult or confusing, ask whether your local hospital has patient advocates, such as those used by the Mayo Clinic (Patient Care at www .patientcare4u.com). Medical Billing Advocates of America (www.billadvocates.com) is another resource that allows you to find an advocate in your state.

For patients contemplating an elective surgery or admission, educate yourself about hospital charges ahead of time—you may find ways to minimize fees for your upcoming hospitalization. Will the hospital accept recent blood tests, EKG, or a chest X-ray done at your doctor's office rather than repeat the tests themselves? Does your hospital charge less when you share a room? Do they offer discounts to uninsured patients? Is it better to be admitted early in the week so you don't "waste" time in the hospital over a weekend when less testing is done? Could your procedure be done in an outpatient surgical center rather than the hospital?

Talk to a patient account representative ahead of time. Check if your local hospital has an online charge list (also known as patient price list). Ask your doctor if she has any recommendations to help you save money. Be your own advocate by speaking up.

64. Ask for a hospital discount

As a self-pay patient, you'll be charged full price for everything, at least initially.

Don't take that as your final answer.

The amount a doctor or hospital charges has little bearing on what they are paid, other than to say the posted charge is the maximum they *might* get paid.

For example, a doctor may charge $100 for an office visit and be reimbursed $65 by Medicare. One private insurance plan may pay $75, another $100, a third only $62 while Medicaid may reimburse a mere $50. In a sense self-pay patients and traditional insurance subsidize plans that underpay. This system is not sustainable in the long run, but for the moment, *your* cost is our concern.

Speak to a patient account representative before hospital admission if you can, or as soon as possible thereafter, and ask for a discount. Read #54 before you go, or take this book with you.

Hospitals use current federal poverty-level guidelines to determine eligibility for discounted fees. For example, the 2010 federal poverty level (FPL) for a family of two is $14,570 or $22,050 for a family of four. At my local hospital, families earning up to twice this may qualify for a 100 percent discount of hospital fees. At three times the poverty level the discount is about 50 percent, tapering off to a 30 percent discount for incomes at 400 percent of FPL. Discounts vary from hospital to hospital, and may apply to outpatient as well as inpatient treatment. If you have the opportunity, research your options before your hospital admission. You will need to complete an application for financial assistance through the hospital. For a complete listing of current federal poverty guidelines, visit the U.S. Department of Health and Human Services Web site at: http://aspe.hhs.gov/POVERTY/09poverty.shtml.

Federal law requires *every* state to offer a Disproportionate Share Hospital (DSH) program, to ensure that low-income and uninsured patients have access to hospital care. Participating hospitals receive government payments to subsidize the cost of unreimbursed hospital-level care to low-income patients. Ask your local hospital about the DSH program in your state. Some states list their hospitals that qualify for DSH online.

Family Size	Federal Poverty Guidelines Discount	Income Limit for 100% Discount	Income Limit for 50% Discount	Income Limit for 30%
1	$10,830	$21,660	$32,490	$43,320
2	$14,570	$29,149	$43,710	$58,280
3	$18,310	$36,620	$54,930	$73,240
4	$22,050	$44,100	$66,150	$88,200

Sample Income Levels for Hospital Discounts Based on Federal Poverty Guidelines

The above is only an example. Discounts will vary according to your state and hospital.

Even if you don't qualify for any of the above discounts, you could still save money with a Prompt Pay Discount. As with any business, the longer a bill goes unpaid, the harder it is to collect. Knowing this, some hospitals have begun offering significant discounts for payment made prior to, or within 30 days of, receiving a service. My local hospital offers a 20 percent Prompt Pay Discount. If yours doesn't advertise this discount, go ahead and ask. Perhaps you'll be pleasantly surprised. If you don't have the cash to pay up front, you might save money by using a credit card, as long as you can pay it off within a year and your interest rate is low. Many hospitals don't charge interest on outstanding bills, however, so if your credit card interest rate is high and you cannot pay off your balance promptly, it might be better to owe the hospital.

Another concept most patients aren't familiar with is that of Diagnosis Related Groups, or DRGs. When a Medicare patient enters the hospital, the hospital is paid a set amount based on the patient's diagnosis. It doesn't matter what the bill is, the hospital gets the same amount whether the patient stays three days or five. Many insurance companies pay hospitals on the same basis. Self-pay patients, however, are charged "à la carte"—per individual item or treatment. If you are self-pay, you might ask whether your hospital bill could be adjusted to whatever the DRG payment for your diagnosis is, often significantly less.

65. Limit the length of your hospital stay

Most patients don't realize they have some control over the length of their hospital stay. But to do so, you need to understand the system.

Sometimes it may seem like you're a patient in the hospital when you're really not. Keep it that way if at all possible. "Outpatient observation" is a period of time, usually under 24 hours, when (though you may be lying in a hospital bed) you haven't been officially admitted to the hospital. If you remain an outpatient, you can save a wad of cash.

Outpatient observation costs considerably less than hospital admission for several reasons. *Over* 24 hours incurs two days of room charges (usually), two days of physician visits, two sets of paperwork. A "23-hour short-term observation" cuts that by half or more, and lessens the administrative cost of a full admission. The specifics may vary from hospital to hospital, and the length of observation may even be extended beyond 23 hours, but the gist of the idea is to remain an outpatient.

Doctors are encouraged to make use of outpatient observation when they're unsure whether a full admission is required. Giving a patient a little time to respond to treatment often clarifies the nature and extent of disease. A 23-hour observation period can always be changed to a full hospitalization if the illness proves more serious than initially suspected. But if you're doing well, you'll be on your way home, where you can recover in the comfort of your own environment. Health problems where short-term observation may be a reasonable alternative to full hospital admission include:

- Abdominal pain
- Acute anxiety or depression
- Asthma attack (or COPD)
- Back pain
- Chest pain other than heart attack
- Dehydration
- Gastroenteritis (stomach flu)
- Headache
- Irregular heart beat (arrhythmia)
- Kidney stone

- Soft-tissue infection
- Urinary tract infection

If your doctor thinks you need to be admitted to the hospital, ask whether a short-term outpatient observation period might be considered. If you improve, or at least don't worsen, perhaps you can leave and follow up with your doctor at his or her office in a day or two. You'll save a bundle and can even sleep in your own bed.

If you *are* admitted to the hospital, realize that half a day may count as a whole, just like prepaid parking. Find out how your hospital calculates daily room-rate charges. Does the day begin at midnight? At noon? Is it the same for everyone, or calculated individually, according to your official time of admission? Ask a social worker or patient account representative how partial days are billed. Will one extra hour be billed as an additional day? If you're paying your own way, you'll want to know: has it been 23 hours or 25? Don't get stuck with an additional $1,000 room charge if a little advance planning is all it takes.

If daily room charges are billed according to your time of admission, ask your nurse what time that was. Don't count on your doctor knowing this. When it's nearing time for your hospital discharge, remind your doctor that you'd like to be released before you are charged for an additional day. Remind your nurse as well, since there's always an extra hour or two of paperwork after your doctor says you can leave.

If you're paying your own way, you'll want to spend as few days in the hospital as possible without jeopardizing your health care. Hospitals start their discharge planning the same day you're admitted to the hospital, and so should you. Once your condition is stabilized, ask your doctor if there's any way your treatment may be continued as an outpatient. Avoid weekends, which are often down times when services such as physical therapy may be unavailable.

There are circumstances when it may cost you less to stay *in* the hospital an extra day or so. If your income qualifies you for a full hospital discount (see #64), and if you are being seen by resident physicians whose services are included in your hospital charges (as opposed to private physician charges, which are billed separately), you may not have any doctor bills to pay. Outpatient visits to your private physician may end up costing you more out of pocket than you'd owe for inpatient physician services.

66. Refuse unnecessary testing and treatment

A big problem with hospital bills is that no one knows what anything costs. Patients don't, nurses don't, doctors don't. Health care workers aren't trained to think that way. They're trained to do "whatever is best for the patient" without regard to cost.

Yet much of what is provided as part of hospital care is not strictly necessary. Certainly, self-pay patients want to eliminate unnecessary extras. But even insured patients and those on Medicare or Medicaid could lower the overall cost of health care services if they were more aware of certain charges.

Over the years I've seen hundreds of patients with oxygen tubing dangling loosely below their noses. If a self-pay patient knew he was paying $150 a day for oxygen (that wasn't even being administered effectively) would he be happy? The doctor himself may have no idea whether the patient is being charged daily or according to actual use. Certainly, patients with heart or lung problems benefit from supplemental oxygen, but it is often ordered routinely in circumstances where it provides no defined benefit.

Or what about paying $150 a day to keep an oxygen monitor on your finger that makes little if any impact on your treatment or recovery? Because the technology exists it becomes the standard of care. But I remember medicine before pulse oximetry was invented. It's a wonderful improvement for patients who would otherwise need arterial blood gas testing, but that doesn't mean everybody needs it.

The cost of having a respiratory therapist administer a breathing treatment or handheld inhaler can easily be $100 per session. If you bring your own inhaler from home or know how to use the one the hospital provides, you may be able to avoid this charge as well.

Another treatment of questionable benefit to a number of patients is patient-controlled analgesia. After surgery patients are commonly connected to an IV pump with pain medicine they can dose themselves. Many patients love this option. Then there are those like me. After my last cesarean, I was ordered such a device, which I found entirely useless. If I ever have surgery again, I will refuse this treatment. If needed, I'll request a pain shot.

You have a right to question tests or treatments you doubt

will benefit you. Asking the nurse why a test or treatment is being done will likely yield the answer, "Because the doctor ordered it." Merely refusing an item, say oxygen, may not remove it from your bill. You or the nurse will need to ask the doctor to write an order to discontinue the service.

Because the history obtained from patients is not always reliable, doctors (especially ones who don't know you) may order tests you believe are unnecessary, such as pregnancy tests and drug screens. You may not even be aware the test has been ordered yet find it on your bill. Other tests, such as a urinalysis or EKG, are often ordered routinely. If you don't understand how a particular test is related to your problem, speak up. Your doctor may be willing to skip it (or the billing department may be willing to drop the charges). This is not to say you should forgo medical tests or procedures that are truly needed. But you need to be your own advocate, since it's unlikely anyone else is watching your wallet.

67. Should you use a teaching hospital?

Your doctor wants to admit you to the hospital. You're sick, scared, and worried about the cost. What should you do?

Of course you want your own doctor, someone you know and trust, to see you through your illness.

But you may save money by seeing a hospital-employed physician at a teaching hospital.

Though a nonteaching hospital may discount your *hospital* fees (see #64), it is unlikely that the *professional* component of your care will be discounted, that is, your doctor bills. Unlike hospitals that receive subsidies to provide charity care, discounts from private fee-for-service doctors are from the goodness of their own hearts.

But professional fees from *hospital-employed physicians* at a teaching hospital will likely fall under the same sliding scale discount policy as hospital fees. The less your income, the less you pay. Bottom line, your total out-of-pocket expenses will be less.

But what is a teaching hospital?

Teaching hospitals teach. They employ resident physicians who are learning aspects of medical treatment beyond that taught in medical school. Experienced physicians oversee the care provided by resident physicians.

Teaching hospitals also usually have various students working with their patients, for example, medical students, student nurses, and X-ray technicians in training.

Does this mean you'll receive inferior care?

No, in fact, teaching hospitals often have the most advanced technology and specialty care, especially if they're affiliated with a medical school.

Receiving care from a teaching hospital does not mean the actual hospital bill will be less. It may be more! There is a degree of inefficiency in the learning process. Physicians unfamiliar with you personally may well order more tests than your family doctor might. But if your income qualifies you for free hospital care, this is not an issue for you.

Private doctors do not receive payment from the hospital for your care. They must submit their own bills in order to get paid. Physician charges for a weeklong stay in the hospital can easily amount to thousands of dollars.

However, being a patient on the "house service" at a hospital means you will be under the care of hospital-employed resident physicians rather than your personal physician. If your income qualifies you for free hospital care, it usually qualifies you for free care from the resident physicians.

Not sick yet? Good. Find your local teaching hospital before you are, so you can head there should you ever need to.

68. Avoid a dozen different doctors

You're admitted to the hospital for a simple hernia.

Your EKG is a little off, so your surgeon consults a cardiologist. He notices your sugar is a bit elevated so calls in an endocrinologist. The endocrinologist worries diabetes may have affected your eyes, but good news!—the ophthalmologist says your eyes are fine, just allergic. When you tell the allergist your back is aching from lying in bed so long, she summons the orthopedist. Lucky for you, your bones look good—could be your kidneys. The urologist says no, perhaps it's your prostate. The ultrasound is OK, but the gastroenterologist advises a colonoscopy.

You beg for a psychiatrist before the doctors drive you crazy.

It sounds ridiculous, but many hospitalized patients hop aboard the specialist merry-go-round without even knowing they've bought a ticket. Each consult generates additional charges, often substantial ones.

And once you're on the merry-go-round it's *very* difficult to get off. Better to avoid the problem in the first place.

Save money—a lot of money—by avoiding having too many doctors.

This applies to insured and uninsured patients alike. It's easier to achieve as an outpatient than an inpatient, but it is possible.

Start by asking your primary care doctor or hospitalist to consult *you*, the patient, *before* consulting other doctors. It's your money, after all. Family docs, internists, and pediatricians are all "specialists" who are also "generalists." They can take care of most bodily afflictions. You don't need a little toe doctor (a super-subspecialist) if you happen to stub it on the bedpost.

Keep in mind other specialists and subspecialists tend to refer to each other. They don't want to step on each other's toes. A cardiologist could treat your elevated blood sugar but usually won't. However, your primary care doctor could interpret your EKG, treat your blood sugar, defer an eye exam until after your hospitalization, treat your allergies, and give you something for your back. Sounds like a bargain!

Ideally, before you need to enter the hospital, you already have a primary care physician who knows you well—a family doctor, an internist, or a pediatrician. And ideally, this same doctor is the one to take care of you in the hospital. Usually a particular problem triggers the need for hospitalization, pneumonia perhaps, or a heart condition. For such a problem, your doctor may well want to consult one additional physician, but it's unlikely you need half a dozen. Suggest to your personal physician that you'd like him or her to take care of you as much as possible, without involving a lot of other doctors. You probably don't need an endocrinologist for your diabetes when your internist has taken care of it for a decade already. The key to this is having a good relationship with your doctor—all the more reason to nurture the relationship (see #2 and #3).

One problem with the above suggestion is that a number of outpatient doctors no longer visit the hospital, referring instead to a "hospitalist" or other physician who spends a lot of time at the hospital. Hospitalist physicians are a newer specialty of doctors who see patients only in the hospital. As the length of hospital stays has decreased, the intensity of hospital treatment has increased, making it difficult for outpatient doctors to keep up with the needs of their hospitalized patients. Another issue is efficiency. It makes little sense for a doctor to travel to the hospital to see one or two patients in the time he could see five times as many at the office. Over the past decade, more and more outpatient doctors have opted to refer their inpatients to hospital-based doctors. Over the years I've come to view my job as keeping patients *out* of the hospital.

Before you need to be hospitalized, ask your doctor what arrangements she would make in case you need hospital care. Hopefully, she would refer you to a doctor she'd be willing to see herself. If you are admitted to the hospital, talk to your primary hospital doctor (the one whose name is on your wristband) and explain that you'd like to limit hospital consults to only those that are strictly necessary.

If you end up seeing several doctors while hospitalized, all of whom schedule follow-up visits afterward, consult your primary care physician as to whether the specialist appointments are truly necessary. Once a specialist has seen you, she may feel an obligation to follow through with your care. If you are transferring all of your care back to your family doctor, please let the specialist know—don't just skip an appointment. If you do need to follow up with a specialist, ask how soon your care can revert to your primary physician.

Try to limit how many doctors you have. It will save thousands in the long run.

69. Avoid duplicate tests

It happens every day. Someone ends up in the hospital and undergoes the same tests we just did a week before.

Patients rarely complain about this because they don't know it's happened, they have little control over the situation, they don't see an itemized bill, and they're not the ones paying.

But those of you who *are* paying won't want to pay for the same test twice.

Of course, at times it *will* be necessary, in order to follow the course of a disease. A blood count two weeks ago may have little bearing on today's pneumonia.

But a thyroid test or HgA1C that was normal last week doesn't need to be repeated this week. An MRI done a month ago may not bear repeating this month if your symptoms haven't changed. A tetanus shot won't need to be administered if you just had one two years ago. You won't need another urine culture if your doctor received culture results a day ago.

So far there is no universal system to transmit health information among various providers. For now, photocopies of relevant records are as quick and reliable as any computer system. And fortunately, you can make your own file and have the information available for any doctor you see. Whenever you have a test done as an outpatient, ask for a copy of the result. You may also want to obtain copies of major tests performed while hospitalized. (You do not need a record of every single blood test performed during a hospital stay, however.)

Start a file of every test you've undergone, organized according to condition and/or date, including:

- Blood work
- Breathing tests
- Cardiac catheterization reports
- CAT scans
- Echocardiograms
- EEGs
- EKGs
- Holter monitor reports
- MRI scans
- Stress test results
- Ultrasounds
- Urine testing
- X-rays

Also include the following in your file:

- Current list of all your medical problems
- List of all prior surgeries and significant injuries

- Current list of all medications, including OTC drugs and herbs
- Current list of all drug allergies and intolerances, including reactions
- List of all hospitalizations, including dates, reasons, and hospital names
- List of all immunizations and TB tests, including dates
- Living will and/or power of attorney
- Contact information for next of kin (whom to contact in case of emergency)
- Names of personal physicians with phone numbers and addresses

70. Have a holiday with that hernia repair

You'd rather take a vacation than spend your hard-earned money on surgery.

Why not do both? *Medical tourism*, as it's called, involves traveling to a country other than your own to receive care.

No one bats an eye when patients from foreign countries seek medical care in the United States. *Why wouldn't they?* Our medical care is the best in the world. But you'll meet with raised eyebrows if you mention going overseas for elective surgery.

Yet for a fraction of what you'd be charged in the United

States you can travel overseas, undergo elective surgery, *and* enjoy a holiday. Some insurance companies have even begun offering their members the option of elective surgery overseas.

In 2008 the AMA adopted a set of guidelines for patients going overseas for care. In brief, overseas care should be voluntary (not mandated by insurance companies looking to cut costs); follow-up care should be assured; legal concerns should be addressed before traveling; patients should seek care at institutions accredited by recognized international entities; financial incentives should not restrict treatment alternatives; and patients should have access to provider licensing and credentials.

Research your options thoroughly, and then talk with your doctor. Don't be surprised, though, if your doctor knows less than you about what's available. Still, your physician should have a good idea about pre-op and post-op concerns, safety issues regarding air travel afterward, and possible complications.

Medical tourism is certainly not for everyone. I'm not even sure it would be for me! But it is a potential way to save money on hospital expenses.

For articles on medical tourism, visit the following sites and do a search for "medical tourism":

American Medical Association: www.ama-assn.org/amed news

Deloitte Center for Health Solutions: www.deloitte.com

Doing an online search for medical tourism Web sites will yield an abundance of results. Two sources that appear reliable are:

WorldMedAssist

www.worldmedassist.com (866) 999-3848

(accredited by the Better Business Bureau)

Companion Global Health Care, Inc.

www.companionglobalhealth care.com (800) 906-7065

(based in Columbia, South Carolina)

CHAPTER EIGHT

Save Money on Ancillary Services

71. Goodwill wheelchairs

You can pay pennies on the dollar for medical equipment. I've been a bargain hunter ever since my grandmother introduced me to the local salvage stores. My exam tables are from Goodwill. My spare wheelchair is from a yard sale.

Perfectly serviceable medical supplies are in abundance. Use your imagination and search them out. Why buy new when something used will work just as well—and cost a lot less?

Look for bargains on medical equipment at:

- Goodwill and Salvation Army stores
- Church and school rummage sales
- Neighborhood sales
- Hospital auxiliary sales
- Local classified ads
- Thrift shops
- Consignment shops

- Salvage freight stores
- Estate and moving sales
- Auctions
- eBay
- www.craigslist.org

Examples of used items you may find include:

- Manual and electric wheelchairs
- Battery-powered scooters
- Crutches
- Walkers
- Manual and electric hospital beds
- Bedside commodes
- Lift chairs
- Shower chairs
- Electric stair climbers
- Medical exercise equipment

Certain items you're probably better off purchasing new, such as those that may be contaminated or require technical maintenance.

Medical items that *require* a prescription theoretically should not be resold, though many are. Some items that patients acquire *with* a doctor's prescription (so that insurance, Medicare, or Medicaid will pay) do not actually require a prescription, including most items on the above list.

Happy hunting.

72. Home breathing treatments

The same breathing treatments you receive at the hospital for asthma or chronic obstructive pulmonary disease (COPD) can be given at home—and *a lot* cheaper.

It isn't the treatments that are so expensive—it's having a team of medical professionals on hand in case the problem worsens.

It's possible to learn your body's signals and treat yourself at home, at least much of the time. Such a plan must be discussed with your doctor, who will be happy to help keep you out of the hospital and away from the ER.

Asthma and COPD make it difficult to breathe, especially to exhale (breathe out). One of the most useful tools to monitor your breathing is a peak flow meter, which measures your ability to exhale effectively. You can buy one online for under $20, or at your local pharmacy. Some insurance will pay for the meter if your doctor writes it as a prescription.

Your doctor will help you establish your normal peak flow and determine levels where it's safe to treat yourself at home, and when you should seek professional medical attention.

To treat yourself at home, you'll need a nebulizer to administer the aerosols. Your doctor can write a prescription to obtain one locally or you can buy one online. (Insurance usually covers the device, which can run $50 to $100 for your initial investment.) Plug-in models are standard but battery-powered devices exist as well. If you can't find one locally, check an online pharmacy such as www.drugstore.com.

You'll also need a prescription for medication. The most common bronchodilators (albuterol solution and ipratropium bromide solution) are on the $4 list (25 single-dose vials for $4, 75 for $10). Bring a copy of the list with you when you request a prescription (see #16 and appendix 4).

These bronchodilators are the same as those in the smaller handheld inhalers, but for a patient having difficulty breathing, the nebulizer treatments seem to allow the medicine to penetrate better.

The medicines are, in themselves, not especially dangerous when used according to directions, *but waiting too long to seek medical attention can be very dangerous, even life-threatening.* Make sure you follow the plan developed by your physician. A home nebulizer can save you money on hospital breathing treatments and ER visits, but not if you use it unwisely.

73. Eyeglasses and contact lenses

Even people with good health insurance may have no coverage for glasses or contact lenses.

Fortunately, there are several ways to lower your costs for eyeglasses, and a few for contact lenses.

Of course, you could start with the large chain stores, which buy in bulk and offer substantial discounts. It's hard to beat their prices.

But the independent optometrist or optician in your community would appreciate your business and may be willing to match chain store discounts *and* give you more personalized service. Tell your local eye doctor that you are self-pay, and ask about affordable options or discounts. Single lens glasses (frames plus lenses) should be available for about $100 and bifocals for under $200.

Save more by keeping your old frames and just getting new lenses if your vision has changed—or vice versa, if your frames are broken. Single-vision lenses (without frames) run about $69, bifocals (with a line) about $129, trifocals about $169, and progressive lenses about $198. Frames alone cost about $80. Though the package deals (frames plus lenses) are a better bargain overall, if you don't have an extra $40 or more to spare, just purchase the single component that you need.

Scattered programs exist to help the needy afford eyeglasses. If your income is less than the federal poverty guidelines ($1,766 a month for a family of four), visit New Eyes for the Needy at www.neweyesfortheneedy.org or call 1-973-376-4903. To participate in this program you must work through a social service agency or school nurse, who can obtain a voucher for you to receive a basic pair of glasses from your local participating optician. The optician then receives payment directly from New Eyes. You must have a prescription for glasses to participate in this program, but on their Web site they list resources by state to help you receive an eye exam at a reduced fee. Also, if you have an old pair of glasses you can't use, send them to New Eyes for the Needy, which will recycle them to a third world country.

Another option is your local Lions Club. Since 1925 Lions

Clubs have helped those in need of eye care but lacking the funds. To find a Lions Club in your area, visit www.lionsclubs .org. They, too, accept used glasses for recycling.

OneSight (at www.onesight.org) works in association with the Lions Clubs and other nonprofit agencies (United Way, Boys and Girls Clubs, homeless shelters, Veterans' Affairs, and others) to provide help for needy patients in North America and throughout the world. They help facilitate the procurement of free glasses from local retail outlets, including LensCrafters, Pearle Vision, Sears Optical, and Target Optical. OneSight also offers regional clinics throughout North America as well as the OneSight Vision Vans, which travel across the United States providing free eye exams and glasses to thousands of children in need.

Some state programs offer children free eye exams and glasses, for example, Florida's Vision Quest. The U.S. Department of Health and Human Services has a Web site, www .insurekidsnow.gov, that lists a program in every state for uninsured children age 18 and under in families earning up to $44,500 (for a family of four). Call 1-877-KIDS-NOW for more information.

As for contact lenses, there are numerous online sites offering free trials and discounted pricing. Again, your local eye center may be willing to price match *and* supply you with a free pair of contacts in case of emergency *and* offer simple eyeglass repairs *and* free eyeglass refittings for customers. Some may also offer a 10 to 33 percent discount on contacts ordered in yearly amounts. Support your community and check locally first.

**Web sites with offers for free or
discounted contact lenses:**

www.acuvue.com

www.allaboutvision.com/premiums

www.bausch.com

www.coopervision.com

www.goodbyereaders.com

---

74. Dental discounts

Are you afraid of your dentist? Afraid of the drill or afraid of the bill?

The cost of routine dental care seems to have outstripped the cost of routine medical care. My charges as a family physician are significantly lower than those of the dentists in the community. In large part this is due to regulation of doctors' fees by Medicare and insurance plans, factors that have left dentists largely unscathed due to the lower number of patients with dental insurance.

Self-pay patients generally pay more than insured patients for dental care. If you have dental insurance, in all likelihood your insurance company has "negotiated" a discount with your provider. (The "negotiation" is usually one-sided, a take-it-or-leave-it offer from the insurance company.) The self-pay patient is left to pay full price.

Finding discounts is a challenge. However, for those of you lacking dental insurance, here are a few ideas you can try.

Ask your dentist for a billing discount. Dentists usually expect self-pay patients to pay on the day of service, yet payment for insured patients requires billing and paperwork (and usually a discount as well). That's worth at least five bucks.

Ask your dentist for a multiple procedure discount. When doctors perform two procedures on the same day, the second procedure is often discounted, on the order of 25 to 50 percent. That's because the time and overhead are less for a single longer visit than for two shorter visits. The same is true of dentists, although they don't automatically offer a discount. But logically, if your dentist has to numb you only once for three fillings instead of three separate visits, it should cost less.

Check with your state dental association. Some state dental associations list programs offering free or reduced-cost services for low-income residents in need of dental care. The Dental Guide USA Web site at www.dentalguideusa.org has links to state dental associations as well as state dental assistance programs.

Try a dental school. Dental schools have affiliated clinics that offer discounted fees based on income. See the American Dental Association's Web site for a list of dental schools at www.ada.org (look under *Education and Careers*).

Visit a Community Health Center. Community Health Centers, located in every state, receive government subsidies to provide medical and dental care to lower-income citizens.

Visit the U.S. Department of Health and Human Services *Find a Health Center* Web site to find a center in your area: www.findahealthcenter.hrsa.gov.

Consider dental tourism. Just as medical tourism is catching on (see #70), dental tourism has become an option for the adventuresome. Read about dental tourism at:

Companion Global Dental (www.companionglobaldental .com)

Discover Medical Tourism (www.discovermedicaltourism .com)

75. Physical therapy versus chiropractic

Bad back? Sore muscles? Stiff neck? Hurting shoulder?

There's more to health care than pills. Hands-on medicine is effective and often preferable, especially in patients who cannot tolerate drugs.

Both physical therapists and chiropractors offer hands-on help with physical ailments.

For those of you *with* insurance, one or the other modality (physical therapy versus chiropractic) may cost you substantially less. Check your benefits for guidance in your decision making, and ask your physician for a referral or recommendations.

For those *without* insurance, the bill for hands-on therapy is easily $50 to $100 a session, likely cost-prohibitive at two or three sessions a week. But there are ways to save.

First, although a few months of therapy may have been

prescribed, you can save hundreds, perhaps thousands of dollars by transitioning to a home exercise program more quickly. Be diligent in your exercises, pay close attention, explain your financial concerns, and work out a plan to meet your needs with the minimum of expense.

Second, before you commit to a program, ask about self-pay discounts or check online. Many physical therapy groups offer 30 to 50 percent discounts for self-pay patients, but most expect payment at the time of services.

Third, you may be eligible for free services. Physical therapy programs affiliated with hospitals may fall under their guidelines for patient discounts (see #64 and #67). Some hospitals may offer discounted physical therapy on a sliding scale basis to uninsured patients with incomes up to 400 percent of the federal poverty level. Talk to a patient financial services representative at your local hospital to find what services you may be eligible to receive at discounted rates.

Lastly, chiropractors sometimes offer a free initial consult and/or X-rays. Some sponsor coupons in regional Entertainment books or phone books. Check your book or check online for details. But remember, there's no free lunch. The goal of any free offer is to convert you to a paying customer. Still, an initial free consult would help you determine whether you're comfortable with the doctor and give you the opportunity to ask the cost of future services. Don't forget to ask whether any discount is available for self-pay or low-income patients.

76. Hearing tests and hearing aids

If you're reading this section, odds are you think you have a hearing problem or know someone who does, or perhaps you need a hearing test for work or for school.

Hearing tests can be administered by your family physician, a specialist, or a private audiologist, or at a hearing aid store. Medical insurance normally covers a hearing test (audiometry) with a prescription from your physician. If you're not insured, consider a free test from a hearing aid store (which may try to sell you a hearing aid).

Or for a general idea of your hearing ability, try one of the free online hearing tests.

- A test much like an audiogram you would receive from your doctor is available from Lloyds at: www.lloyd hearingaid.com/audiogram_start.cfm. You will derive the most benefit from this test if you follow the online instructions regarding background noise elimination.

- Although this site is complex, demonstrating equal loudness contours, it allows you to graph your hearing across a wide spectrum of frequencies. Please follow the instructions carefully at: www.phys.unsw.edu.au/ jw/hearing.html.

- For a very simple test, visit www.freehearingtest.com. You should be able to hear every tone on the five-tone test. This site also allows you to listen to environmental sounds and features an audio download to explain and experience simulated hearing loss, as well as tinnitus.

- To evaluate your hearing in the presence of back-ground noise, take the Phonak Hearing Test, which simulates the problem people have with age-related hearing loss: www.phonak.com/phonak/com/b2c/en/hearing/recognizing_hearingloss/hearingtest.html.

If you need a hearing aid, look before you leap. Hearing loss is rarely an emergency and you have time to shop around and compare. Special offers are rarely one-time opportunities.

The cost of a single hearing aid is somewhere between $500 and $5,000, which is *not* covered by Medicare. Since private insurance often *does* pay for a hearing aid, it's a good idea to get your hearing checked *before* you reach Medicare age.

If You'll Be the One Paying, Check Out These Resources First

- Miracle-Ear offers free hearing aids to children of lower-income families. Contact them at: www.miracleear.com/childrenrequest.aspx.
- Starkey Hearing Foundation offers free hearing aids for low-income adults and children without other resources. Income guidelines vary according to family size, beginning at $18,403 for an individual, up to $37,221 for a family of four. An application may be downloaded at their Web site, www.sotheworldmayhear.org/hearnow/, or call 1-800-328-8602.
- Lions Clubs International offers assistance to hearing-impaired individuals. Request help at:

www.lionsclubs.org/EN/our-work/sight-programs/
assistance-requests.php.
- The Let Them Hear Foundation offers services and
hearing aids for those with inadequate resources at:
www.letthemhear.org/default.php.

If you're an employed adult or one seeking employment, check your local Vocational Rehabilitation office, which may assist with the procurement of a hearing aid on the basis of employment rehabilitation.

New and used hearing aids are for sale on eBay and elsewhere, but use caution and common sense when purchasing any used medical device.

77. Mental health

The cost of mental health care goes beyond that of seeing a physician and buying medicine. Lost work, missed school, alcoholism, child abuse or neglect, and family disruption all add to the cost of mental illness.

And though health insurance usually covers treatment of mental illness, limitations are common, and many patients remain uninsured. However, as of July 1, 2010, this is changing, at least for group insurance plans for businesses with more than 50 employees. They will no longer be able to set higher co-pays or deductibles, nor enforce stricter limits for mental illness, nor are they permitted to establish separate deductibles for mental and physical illnesses. With time this change will likely broaden to include smaller group and individual insurance plans.

In the meantime—regardless of insurance—good news: help is available.

Start with your family doctor, who may prescribe medication, provide counseling, or refer you for additional services. As a family physician, I treat depression, anxiety, and life-related stress on a daily basis, often choosing medications that cost as little as $4 a month. Bring a copy of a $4 list from your local discount pharmacy with you when you go for an appointment (see #16).

If you need one of the more expensive medications, read #18 to learn about patient assistance programs. Read all of chapter 2 for more ideas on how to save money on prescription medications.

Next, consider the resources your community has to offer. If your local college or university has a psychology department, they likely have an affiliated clinic that offers free or discounted counseling services. If your local hospital is a teaching hospital (one with resident physicians), it should offer clinics where you can see a medical or psychiatric resident physician at a reduced charge.

If you feel comfortable with your pastor or other religious leader, talk to him or her about your problems. Counseling abilities vary, and it's legitimate to ask what training or experience he or she may have in the field. A trusted teacher or wise friend may serve as well when your concerns are those common to the human condition—family, job, and friends.

For professional help, ask your local community health center about medical and counseling services. Some centers offer free or discounted medication as well. Check your local health department, likewise. If they don't have a program to assist you, they should know who does. For additional information about depression and community health centers, read #34.

The U.S. Department of Health and Human Services Substance Abuse and Mental Health Administration's Web site lists over a dozen hotlines for various problems including suicide prevention, child abuse, missing children, and domestic violence. For a list of National Toll-Free Help Lines, see: www.mentalhealth.samhsa.gov/hotlines.

For specific hotlines according to condition or problem, visit the Health Hotlines Subject Index at: http://healthot lines.nlm.nih.gov/subserch.html.

Mental health resources according to state of residence are available as well at: http://mentalhealth.samhsa.gov.

Lastly, if you're in the midst of crisis and need help now, call the National Crisis Hotline at 1-800-273-8255 (TTY 1-800-799-4889).

78. Exercise versus physical therapy

Money talks. It talks people into exercising. When 1,000 bucks of therapy is on the line, people find it easier to get off the couch and get moving.

Although professional guidance is helpful, physical therapy is expensive. For a self-pay patient, it could easily run beyond the cost of a year's utilities.

Physical therapy (PT) isn't magic—it's mainly stretching,

strengthening, and retraining muscles in a controlled environment, with professional instruction and supervision. If you're careful, you can save big bucks by doing your own rehab.

Common reasons for referral to physical therapy include:

- Low-back pain
- Neck pain or stiffness
- Shoulder pain or stiffness
- Sciatica or hip pain
- Deconditioning (being out of shape)
- Imbalance or falling

Most of these conditions are amenable to physical therapy or guided exercise (unless they're severe enough for surgery, or if some other underlying cause is present). A few weeks with a skilled trainer may work wonders. For low-back pain and sciatica, regular walking or swimming, 20–30 minutes, three–five times a week, would be a good start. Some insurance plans are now offering fitness and exercise programs as a paid benefit.

If you have some idea why you're hurting, say you strained your back or shoulder, you may want to try treating yourself at home before consulting your doctor. If you have a problem that starts out of the blue, it's probably better to see your physician first.

If your doctor suggests physical therapy, ask whether a trial of exercise on your own is appropriate. Ask for guidelines on how long to wait before seeking further advice. If you are considering therapy, check whether you have a co-pay on physical therapy sessions, or a limit on the number of visits. If you go to PT, make sure you understand and comply with the home exercise program they recommend both between therapy sessions and after completion of the program.

A selection of trustworthy Web sites with instruction in rehabilitation exercises you can do at home includes:

- www.askthetrainer.com (with videos)
- www.familydoctor.org
- www.mayoclinic.com
- http://my.clevelandclinic.org
- http://nihseniorhealth.gov/exerciseforolderadults/toc.html
- www.shoulder-pain-management.com
- www.sport-fitness-advisor.com
- www.webmd.com

If you don't improve within a few weeks, consult your doctor. If you've saved $1,000, take a relaxing vacation, but don't forget your exercises.

---

79. Lab testing at home

You can save money by testing yourself at home. In these days of consumer demand and exploding technology, an amazing array of home medical devices and tests have become available.

You don't need a doctor's order to check whether you are ovulating, have HIV, diabetes, high cholesterol, or urinary tract infection, are in menopause, or even if you have drugs in your urine.

Many are excellent, cost-effective, and FDA-approved. Others may be scams, so before you buy, check the U.S. Food and Drug Administration's Web site at www.fda.gov, where you can find a link to a database of FDA-approved home lab tests (www.fda.gov/MedicalDevices/ProductsandMedicalProcedures/InVitroDiagnostics/LabTest/ucm126079.htm).

Numerous Web sites offer testing for a variety of other conditions *not* on the above FDA list, claiming FDA approval. This may be true in a sense, since only the specimen is collected at home, then mailed elsewhere for analysis, possibly to an FDA-approved lab.

For example, home DNA paternity testing is offered online (for hundreds of dollars). You collect the specimens, then mail them to a (hopefully accredited) lab. Such tests may be useful for your own information, but without proof of proper collection they won't be accepted as legal evidence.

The FDA's list for home medical tests includes:

- Alcohol breath tests
- Allergy tests
- Blood loss in the stool (occult blood)
- Blood sugar (glucose)
- Cholesterol (total, LDL, HDL)

- Hemoglobin A1C
- HIV/AIDS
- Menopause
- Ovulation
- Pregnancy
- Semen for infertility
- Urinary tract infection
- Urine drug screen
- Specific tests for many other chemicals

Talk to your doctor about the most effective use of these over-the-counter test kits. For example, if you detect blood in your stool, what are the implications? What's the next step? If you test positive for a urinary infection, should you take medication? Does a negative HIV test guarantee you don't have the disease? What does a menopause test imply?

If saving money is your primary concern, remember that many of these tests are available through your local health department or hospital clinic at a reduced cost (see chapters 3, 4, and 6). Ask your doctor how a specific home test can help you lower your medical expenses and help you partner in your own health care.

80. Herbal medicines and supplements

Will the use of herbs and supplements save you money on health care?

In recent years many patients have turned—or better yet, returned—to herbal therapies. It's certainly not a new concept.

A number of our current medications are derived from herbal sources: aspirin, digoxin, narcotics, hormones.

The main problem with herbal therapies is that most have not been studied in large, double-blind placebo-controlled trials—and likely never will be, largely due to cost concerns and lack of FDA regulation. This does not necessarily mean that they are ineffective, but rather that there is little scientific evidence to clarify their role as effective therapies.

Of course, in other cultures, herbal preparations have been used for thousands of years. Experience ought to count for something. But with 30 percent of people responding to *any* therapy—the placebo effect—it's difficult to tell whether the therapy is what's effective, or simply the belief in a particular therapy.

Patients complain about the cost of medication. Yet many spend more—and willingly—on over-the-counter herbs and supplements. According to the July 2009 National Health Statistics Report (www.nccam.nih.gov/news/camstats/costs/nhsrn18.pdf), Americans spend over $33 billion out of pocket annually on visits to complementary and alternative medicine practitioners, product purchases, materials, and classes.

Why the discrepancy in attitude? I believe it's because people want to be in charge of their own bodies. Generally speaking, we'd rather follow our own line of thinking than submit to another person's recommendations. Taking herbs and supplements makes us feel in control, even if we can't perceive a benefit. That's not to say no one receives a benefit, but the majority of my patients who take supplements are unable to express what that benefit has been or might be. Rather, it's some vague, hoped-for improvement.

Some of my patients have the mistaken belief that anything that's natural is safe. I often remind them that poison mushrooms and poison ivy are natural as well, but to partake of them is ill-advised. Certain herbal preparations can interfere or interact with prescription medications, causing side effects beyond those that a natural remedy might cause if taken alone.

Other people distrust the pharmaceutical companies and the health care industry as a whole, citing medications that have been withdrawn from the market, such as Vioxx or Redux. Certainly the practice of medicine is imperfect, and the profit motive sometimes conflicts with what is best for an individual patient.

But it doesn't necessarily follow that those who sell herbal products have superior motives or better evidence for their products. A small scientific study suggesting a possible benefit in select individuals should not be extrapolated to major benefits for a large population.

Like many medical doctors, I commonly prescribe preparations for which scientific studies are available: calcium, certain vitamins, saw palmetto, melatonin, chondroitin sulfate, and glucosamine. I have difficulty recommending others, though cannot say they aren't beneficial.

The problem I see most commonly is that people believe herbal remedies will do more than they can do. If an herbal preparation claims to lower blood sugar, perhaps it's true—to a degree. Maybe it *can* lower your sugar 10 or 20 points. But if your blood sugar is 200 points too high, medication is what you need—likewise with cholesterol and blood pressure. Whereas a mild case of depression or arthritis may respond to St. John's wort or glucosamine, respectively, severe degenerative arthritis and suicidal depression will likely require medication.

Back to the question at hand: will the use of herbs and supplements save you money on health care? The potential savings is twofold. If you use an over-the-counter product and find it is effective, you may be able to avoid both a trip to your doctor and associated fees. On the other hand, if you're spending good money on herbal products month after month and cannot say they've improved your health, it only makes sense to discontinue the ineffective product and keep your money in your pocket.

It is unlikely that using herbs and supplements will save you a significant amount on medication. With the price of generic drugs so low (see #16), it's doubtful that herbal preparations will be any cheaper.

However, if you have arthritis, are intolerant of traditional generic NSAIDs, are uninsured, and are prescribed Celebrex, you might find that taking glucosamine plus chondroitin saves money and provides equivalent relief. Likewise, saw palmetto may be as helpful for prostatic symptoms as certain brand-name prescription drugs, and is available inexpensively over the counter.

Use common sense to spare your pocketbook. If your blood sugar is *a little* high, perhaps chromium will help. If your cholesterol is *somewhat* elevated, garlic (and dietary restrictions) may improve your numbers. If you've got the winter blues, St. John's wort may perk you up.

But while keeping healthy and avoiding the doctor is a laudable goal, if you have clear-cut medical problems, don't rely on herbal products alone. Take your supplements to your doctor and discuss the best course of action. Ask whether it's wise to spend $20 a month on vitamins when you're having trouble affording your diabetic medicine. Think about what you're actually trying to accomplish. Find successful ways to be in charge of your own health care. Don't take an herbal product for a year if it's not helping you. If acupuncture relieves your pain, that's wonderful, and insurance may cover this. But if 20 sessions haven't helped, 40 probably won't either.

The National Center for Complementary and Alternative Medicine (www.nccam.nih.gov, 1-888-644-6226) provides extensive information regarding the wise use of supplements. In its listing of herbal products, NCCAM includes what science says regarding side effects and potential benefits.

The American Academy of Family Physicians makes their medical journal available to the public free of charge at their Web site, www.aafp.org (except for the most recent 12 issues, which require a paid subscription). The site includes many articles on rational use of herbal preparations and supplements. Several articles of interest are listed below:

Is Herbal Therapy Safe in Cardiovascular Disease?

www.aafp.org/afp/2002/1001/p1318.html

Evaluating Perioperative Use of Herbal Medications

www.aafp.org/afp/2002/0501/p1927.html

Is Herbal Tea Effective for Pain of Acute Pharyngitis?

www.aafp.org/afp/2003/1101/p1840.html

Herbal and Dietary Supplements for Treatment of
    Anxiety Disorders

www.aafp.org/afp/2007/0815/p549.html

Herbal Health Products—What You Should Know

www.aafp.org/afp/990301ap/990301e.html

Herbal and Dietary Supplement-Drug Interactions in
    Patients with Chronic Illnesses

www.aafp.org/afp/2008/0101/p73.html

Health Effects of Hawthorn

www.aafp.org/afp/2010/0215/p465.html

Outpatient Management of Anticoagulation Therapy
    (food and herbs that interact with warfarin)

www.aafp.org/afp/2007/0401/p1031.html

CHAPTER NINE

Save Money Using 10 Practical Over-the-Counter Treatments

81. Waste that wart

For decades doctors have used cryotherapy (freezing therapy) to kill warts. Now you can do it yourself and save $50 to $100 in doctor bills.

Traditionally, physicians have used liquid nitrogen to cause a local "frostbite" to a wart, thereby killing it. The warty skin dies off, and normal skin regrows in its place.

The OTC products use propellants (similar to those in hairspray) to accomplish the same goal.

At this writing there are three OTC products available:

- Compound W Freeze Off Wart Removal System
- Dr. Scholl's Freeze Away
- Wartner Wart Removal System

For $11 to $25 you can treat your own wart (or your family member's wart), but there are a few things to keep in mind.

First, these freezing treatments are for common warts (on the hands and elsewhere) and plantar warts (on the feet), but not for genital warts or facial warts due to concerns about scarring.

Second, the treatment is not painless, which is especially of concern with children. Consider the "kinder, gentler" approach using daily salicylic acid applications (e.g., Dr. Scholl's Clear Away).

Third, length of freezing is vital. Too little and the wart grows back between treatments. Too much and scarring may occur. It is difficult for the layperson to know how long to freeze. Follow the package directions, but you may want to err on the side of too little. You can always freeze the wart again in a few days if nothing happens. Even doctors often need to treat a large wart more than once.

Not all warts respond—some grow too quickly, and what you think is a wart might not be. See your doctor if what looks like a wart persists.

For more savings, check product Web sites for coupons and your local drugstore for periodic sales.

82. Calm the carpal tunnel

You type a lot. You've checked the Web sites. You're sure you have carpal tunnel syndrome.

You may be right. Try treating yourself and save an office call.

Carpal tunnel syndrome is very common, especially among those who use their hands and wrists in a repetitive fashion.

Pain, numbness, or tingling in the hand is often caused by pressure on the median nerve as it passes through the "carpal tunnel" inside the wrist. In severe cases there may be weakness as well or even muscle wasting (shrinkage). Conditions associated with water retention, such as pregnancy, may also induce the condition.

There is an easy test to confirm the diagnosis—the symptoms should involve only your first three-and-a-half fingers. The little finger and the outside edge of the ring finger should not be affected. Test yourself when you're having symptoms, and see your doctor if the pattern is otherwise. If the onset of symptoms is sudden, go to the ER—*it could be a stroke!*

Relieving the pressure on the nerve is the mainstay of therapy. Avoiding excess use of the hands and wrists often allows minor swelling to resolve, enough to take pressure off the nerve. Immobilizing the wrist helps. Carpal tunnel splints are available at your local drugstore and online. I suggest looking locally to obtain the best fit.

The splint needs to be comfortable and needs to keep your wrist in the neutral position. If you relax your forearm and hand on the table while seated, with your fingers naturally curved, you'll see what the neutral position should be. It is not completely straight. There should be no pressure points within the splint, which should be snug but not tight.

Some people respond well to wearing the splint during times of hand or wrist usage. Others do well to wear the splint at night, especially pregnant women. It may take weeks of splinting to notice a significant difference. Be patient.

Ice and NSAIDs (nonsteroidal anti-inflammatory drugs— see #96) may help reduce swelling that is producing pressure on the nerve as well, especially if the cause is an acute case of overwork.

Carpal tunnel syndrome may require surgery or cause permanent damage if the pressure on the nerve persists. If these simple treatments don't improve the problem within a month or two, and especially if symptoms are worsening despite these recommendations, see your doctor.

83. Rid the lice

You don't need to see a doctor for head lice.

The most common reasons I see patients for head lice are: 1) they don't know over-the-counter (OTC) treatment is available; 2) they haven't used OTC treatment correctly; or 3) their co-pays on office visits and medications run less than the OTC treatment.

And some people come because they *think* they have head lice but they don't. Usually they have dandruff instead.

Head lice cause itching (but so can other conditions). The lice themselves are difficult to see. The diagnosis is normally made by seeing nits (lice eggs), pearly little ovals that are *stuck* to the hair shaft, commonly within an inch of the scalp. White flakes that are easily dislodged are usually dandruff, not nits (see #98).

You can save money ridding yourself of lice by:

- Using OTC treatment, thus saving an office call
- Calling your doctor, who may prefer to treat you over the phone without seeing you

- Using prescription products if you're lucky enough to have co-pays lower than the $20 the OTC treatment costs

There is ample information online about head-lice prevention and treatment. For comprehensive information about pediculosis capitis (head lice), visit these Web sites:

- For a one-page handout on head lice from the American Academy of Family Physicians: www.aafp.org/afp/20040115/349ph.html.
- For everything you ever wanted to know about head lice, including informative and entertaining videos: National Pediculosis Association Web site: www.headlice.org.
- For concise information in both English and Spanish from the Centers for Disease Control and Prevention: www.cdc.gov/lice.

As for saving money, I suggest using the Rid Lice Elimination System (about $20), which includes the lice-killing shampoo/conditioner, the nit Comb-Out Gel, and the Home Lice Control Spray. Read the directions carefully, re-treat if necessary, and check out the above Web sites for extra tips. For questions related to using Rid (and possibly a coupon), visit their Web site at: www.ridlice.com or call 1-800-RID-LICE (1-800-743-5423). The phone number also features audio instructions regarding lice detection and control.

For patients looking for a natural way to cure lice, several options are available. Hot air has been shown to kill head lice and decrease the hatch rate of louse eggs. According to the medical journal *Pediatrics*, the Lousebuster device is among the most effective. Visit their Web site at www.lousebuster .com or call 1-877-781-0999.

Shaving the head is another option, especially popular with boys. It is not recommended for reluctant children, especially girls, who are resistant to having their heads shorn.

Suffocating the lice is a third option. Research is underway to find the optimum method. Coating the hair and scalp thoroughly with petroleum jelly or other occlusive product may be effective. If you try petroleum jelly, it must be left on at least several hours and probably will need to be repeated as additional eggs hatch.

Lastly, pubic lice (crabs) often respond to the above mentioned treatments . . . applied elsewhere. For scabies (invisible critters) see your doctor.

84. Tape the tear

You've cut yourself and hate to spend hundreds of dollars at the emergency room.

As you stand there bleeding all over the garage, your eyes light on a fresh roll of duct tape. Survivor man that you are, you reach for the forbidden fruit. "Stop," screams your wife. "We're going to the hospital!" But it might have worked, you sigh.

There's no magic in suturing a wound together. Though stitches are the traditional way to close a laceration, other closure techniques work as well, and may save you a trip to the doctor.

Taping is an excellent answer more often than you'd expect. It works well when a wound:

- Is no deeper than skin deep
- Does not gape open
- Runs with the skin lines (the "grain")
- Is not contaminated
- Occurs in someone who will protect the area from further injury for at least five days
- Occurs in an area that the patient is willing and able to keep clean for at least five days

Wound length is also a factor, though I've used the technique successfully on wounds up to three inches long—*but* only where there was no tension across the wound (where it lies nicely together like a seam) *and* only when the injured person was able and willing to protect the area from further injury for several days. Generally, taping works best on wounds no longer than an inch in length.

Active children and active workers are questionable candidates for taping. Sutures and staples are stronger and can hold the deeper tissues together. Also facial injuries usually require professional attention due to cosmetic concerns.

And be sure to get a tetanus shot within 48 hours of the injury if it's been 10 years or longer since your last vaccine.

So, you've sliced your leg with a clean razor knife, you've cleansed the wound with fresh, soapy water, the edges do not gape, and you've decided to tape.

Don't use duct tape . . . get medical tape, such as Nexcare Steri-Strip Skin Closure Adhesive Surgical Tape Strips (for about $10). You have time to go to the drugstore. Bandage yourself first so you don't bleed in public.

Tape yourself neatly together according to package directions—there should be little if any tension across the wound. Applying a topical over-the-counter antibiotic (bacitracin) after taping is a consideration, but it usually prevents the tape from sticking well. Better to clean and dry the wound thoroughly before taping, and to keep it clean and dry afterwards.

Leave the tape on undisturbed at least five days, but check daily for signs of infection (redness, pus, swelling, pain, or odor). If these symptoms occur, see your doctor promptly. If the tapes don't fall off by 10 days, go ahead and remove them. Your wound should be healed by then.

With the $100 you save, buy more first aid supplies—sounds like you'll need them.

85. Band your tennis elbow

The majority of tennis elbow isn't caused by playing tennis.

Sure you can get it from tennis or other racquet sports—especially if your backhand stroke needs some improvement.

But in most patients, repetitive household tasks are much more likely suspects—painting, raking, digging, scraping, wall-papering.

As for occupations, I've seen tennis elbow in plumbers, pipe fitters, roofers, construction workers, bricklayers—any activity that uses the forearm in a repetitive motion. The overuse puts a strain on the tendons of the forearm where they attach to the bone at the outside of the elbow (the lateral epicondyle—hence the name, lateral epicondylitis). A beautiful video of the physiology of tennis elbow may be viewed at: www.youtube.com/watch?v=_JPDwLu9UAI&feature=related.

In many cases you can save a trip to the doctor by treating yourself.

If you perform one of these or a similar repetitive task and your elbow becomes tender and starts to ache, the simplest answer is—rest. Stop whatever activity you suspect is the cause and see if the area improves.

In addition to avoiding overuse, ice and short term use of anti-inflammatory medications such as ibuprofen or naproxen may lessen the symptoms (see #96, the NSAIDs).

The so-called *tennis elbow band* is also useful and is available over the counter for $10 to $20. The intent of the band is to relieve the pressure on the elbow by effectively shortening the tendon. More often than not, though, I've seen these bands used incorrectly. The band needs to be worn about two inches below the elbow, depending on your size, with the pressure point toward the upper, outer edge of the forearm.

Before you apply the band, move your arm to intentionally bring on the discomfort. After applying the band, repeat the same movement. If the discomfort has not improved, adjust the band up or down a bit, or move the pressure point of the band inward or outward. If *you* can't tell if the band makes any difference, odds are it won't.

Exercises for tennis elbow may be found at: www.aafp.org/afp/2007/0915/p849.html.

If the above measures don't resolve the problem within

a few weeks, see your doctor. Tennis elbow may require physical therapy, steroid injection, or even surgery. Occasionally, the problem may be something else entirely, such as bursitis.

86. Taper the tobacco

If you smoke one pack a day for a year, for the amount you spend on cigarettes, you could vacation in Hawaii. At 5 bucks a day, that's over $1,500 a year.

Can't stop cold turkey? Try the nicotine replacement products, now for sale OTC.

Lozenges, gum, and patches are all available without a prescription. In my experience the patches are the most effective aid in smoking cessation. Other methods supply nicotine orally (by mouth), which is too similar to smoking to be effective in many patients.

Nicoderm and Habitrol were both by prescription only when first released. Now, for about the price of half a pack of cigarettes a day, you can obtain them over the counter. Generic patches cost slightly less.

If your problem is nicotine addiction, these products definitely work. If you smoke for other reasons—friends, nerves, habit—you'll need more than a patch to quit. Determination is the primary ingredient. If you are *not* determined to succeed, hold off on using these products until motivation and circumstance make your success more likely. But if you're ready to quit and want to avoid nicotine withdrawal symptoms, the nicotine patches are a proven benefit.

Although you don't need to see a doctor to use these products, there is value in seeing your physician. There are other prescription products that can be used in combination with the patch to improve its effectiveness. Also, committing to checking in with your physician adds the element of accountability to your decision to quit. Of course, you don't need a doctor to hold you accountable. A trusted friend may do as well.

Looking for reasons to quit smoking? According to the Centers for Disease Control and Prevention (CDC), tobacco use causes 5 million deaths worldwide per year, with more than 8 million deaths annually projected by 2030. On average, smokers die 13–14 years younger than nonsmokers. In the United States cigarette smoking is the leading preventable cause of death, accounting for one in five deaths annually.

Of course, most smokers already know that cigarette smoking causes cardiovascular disease, lung disease, and cancer. So what about the cost? If you're reading this book, you must be somewhat concerned. Have you tried one of the online cost calculators such as the one at Health.com, which shows how much you spend on cigarettes? Check it out at: www.health.com/health/library/mdp/0,,calc011,00 .html#calc011-sec for a real eye-opener. A one-pack-a-day habit will easily drain $20,000 from your bank account over the next decade.

The cost to society is staggering. According to the CDC, cigarette smoking costs the United States $193 billion every year, half in lost productivity, half in health care costs. Imagine what good America could do if that money were spent to prevent disease rather than treat it.

For more information on the risks of smoking, visit the CDC's tobacco morbidity and mortality page at: www.cdc.gov/tobacco/data_statistics/fact_sheets/fast_facts/index.htm.

Enjoy the additional benefits of becoming a nonsmoker. Your breath will be fresher, your teeth whiter, your clothes cleaner. You'll breathe easier, food will taste better, your sense of smell will improve.

Quit now and your bottom line will improve along with your health. *Happy breathing!*

The Nicoderm CQ Web site offers the Committed Quitters Program as well as a printable coupon toward their product at: www.nicodermcq.com.

The Habitrol Web site offers the Smoke-Free Program to increase your likelihood of success at: www.habitrol.com/index.html.

---

87. Butcher the bugs

What do doctors and hospitals use to prevent infection in lacerations? The same antibiotic ointment you can find over the counter for $5.

Bacitracin is an excellent drug for prevention and treatment of mild skin infections. Doctors use it more commonly than prescription antibiotic ointments—*because it works.*

Cleaning an open wound, then applying bacitracin may well save you a trip to the doctor for infection.

Examples of injuries and lesions where this antibiotic ointment is appropriate include:

- Abrasions
- Mild road-rash
- Small lacerations
- Lacerations that have been stapled or sutured
- Small burns with superficial blistering
- Diaper rash that appears mildly infected (also see #88)
- Insect bites that appear mildly infected
- Small areas of impetigo
- Injuries near the mouth and nose

Generally the treated area should look better within a day or two. If the affected area is expanding, becomes redder, feels hot to the touch, or develops swelling, pain, or pus, the infection may be deeper and require antibiotics by mouth. See your doctor promptly if this is the case.

Unless a person is known to be allergic, bacitracin can be used preventively by just about everyone. However, it is not necessarily sufficient in babies, diabetics, or people with cancer, swelling, poor circulation, or general poor health.

Triple Antibiotic Ointment is an OTC antibacterial ointment that contains bacitracin in addition to neomycin and polymyxin B. It is generally no better than bacitracin alone and is more likely to cause a skin allergy due to the neomycin.

Bacitracin is also available by prescription as an eye ointment. Should you have this leftover from an eye infection it could be safely used elsewhere on the body, but not vice versa. (Don't use regular OTC bacitracin in the eye.)

Doctors, ERs, and urgent care centers often keep packets of bacitracin on hand and may be willing to give you enough for a small area free of charge, especially if they've seen you for a laceration or abrasion. Whenever you use bacitracin, whether you've seen a physician or not, keep in mind that a worsening infection will likely require a prescription for oral antibiotics.

88. Eradicate the rash

Though most steroid creams remain by prescription only, the 0.5 and 1.0 percent hydrocortisone preparations are available OTC for as little as $4. Used regularly, hydrocortisone is an effective remedy for many common skin conditions including:

- Mild poison ivy
- Allergic skin rashes
- Chemical dermatitis (such as exposure to detergents, soaps, and solvents)
- Mild to moderate eczematous (atopic) dermatitis
- Diaper dermatitis
- Mild idiopathic dermatitis (of unknown cause)
- Sunburn
- Insect bites

Many dry, scaly, itchy rashes respond to hydrating the skin alone—apply a mild skin lotion (such as Keri Lotion) immediately after washing, even before your skin is quite dry. This seals in the moisture and allows the skin to heal. If there's no improvement by a week or so, try applying hydrocortisone cream as well. If symptoms still persist despite daily application, the rash could be a fungus or could require a stronger steroid cream (or other medication), for which you'll need to see your doctor. If you're unsure as to the cause of your rash, there's very little chance that using hydrocortisone cream will cause a problem, and it should not mask a serious condition.

With dishpan hands the skin is usually both dry and irritated. Sometimes using a different brand of dish detergent will make a difference. Try one free of dyes and perfumes. Wearing gloves is sometimes helpful (I use latex-free medical gloves at times). Applying a perfume-free lotion such as Gold Bond Ultimate Healing Skin Therapy Lotion or Vaseline Intensive Rescue *immediately* after exposing your hands to water is very helpful. Cortaid Maximum Strength or generic 1 percent hydrocortisone cream or ointment should help decrease redness and itching as well.

Regarding diaper rash—though the name suggests the diaper as the cause of the rash, this is rarely the case. Although occasionally a child may be sensitive to a particular brand of diapers, usually the problem is a chemical irritation due to prolonged contact with urine or feces. Therefore, frequent diaper changes and keeping the area dry are first-line therapy.

Zinc oxide ointment applied to the diaper area provides an effective barrier to allow sensitive skin to heal. Hydrocortisone cream will lessen the redness and perhaps make the rash more comfortable as well.

A simple diaper rash is usually pink with tiny bumps. Larger bumps and more redness often indicate infection, commonly due to yeast, especially after taking antibiotics for infection elsewhere. Typically yeast diaper dermatitis responds well to antifungal medications such as clotrimazole (available without a prescription). Only occasionally does bacterial infection occur, in which case bacitracin may help. If none of these OTC treatments resolves the rash, consult your doctor.

89. Heal the hemorrhoids

Hurting heinie: Strictly speaking, the heinie is the buttocks. But between the fleshy folds may lurk troublesome hemorrhoids (piles).

A hemorrhoid is a mass of distended, swollen blood vessels around the rectum (similar to varicose veins). In their swollen state, hemorrhoids may be the size of grapes or even plums. In their shrunken state they resemble soft, pink, fleshy raisins or prunes, either inside or outside the anus.

Internal hemorrhoids are located just inside the rectum. They may cause an achy fullness or cause no discomfort at all. Bleeding from internal hemorrhoids is often painless but can be more alarming, enough to turn the toilet water red. Unless a doctor has diagnosed you with internal hemorrhoids, see a physician if bleeding occurs.

External hemorrhoids are more bothersome but generally only bleed enough to streak the BM or stain the toilet tissue. External hemorrhoids are located just outside the rectum, are often tender, and can be detected by the patient. Look in a mirror if you're curious.

Both types of hemorrhoids are associated with constipation or straining (which can occur with diarrhea, too). To avoid developing hemorrhoids, keep your BMs soft by eating a diet high in water-soluble fiber. High-fiber foods include whole grains, fruits, and vegetables. Aim for five servings a day. Another alternative is a bulk laxative such as Metamucil or stool softener such as Surfak.

> See www.metamucil.com/fiber-guide-fruits.php for a listing of higher-fiber foods or www.citrucel.com for a dietary fiber calculator and coupons.

The symptoms of hemorrhoids can usually be treated effectively using OTC remedies. I'm a firm believer in the power of hot baths to shrink swollen hemorrhoids. The water needs to be quite warm to be effective—be careful not to burn yourself. Soaking half an hour or so daily for several days helps as much as any medication—and for free.

OTC medications such as Preparation H contain phenylephrine to shrink swollen hemorrhoids, pramoxine to numb the area, and a soothing lubricant. OTC hydrocortisone 1 percent cream can be used for itching and inflammation.

Prescription medications exist but are basically the same, just stronger (higher dose). Save yourself a pile of money and treat your piles at home. If you're not better in a week or two, consult your doctor.

90. Abolish the acne

Acne treatment can cost anywhere from $10 to well over $1,000!

Fortunately, unless you've got a bad case, you can treat yourself at home using a prescription medicine that's also available over the counter.

For over 50 years, benzoyl peroxide has been a mainstay of acne treatment. It is as effective as many expensive prescription antibiotic creams. To get the most out of the treatment, you need to know a little more about acne.

Acne is more than "oily" skin. Pimples form as a result of skin *inflammation, not infection*. The germ *Propionibacterium acnes* likes to live in hair follicles, where it converts sebum into free fatty acids. These acids are irritating to the human body, which makes "pus" to fight them off, resulting in a blackhead or whitehead, or pimple or pustule.

Benzoyl peroxide does two things: it kills the germ that leads to pimple formation and it helps new skin replace the old. Mostly it works by preventing new pimples from forming while the body heals those already present. There is no overnight treatment for acne, not even by prescription. You can't dab the medicine on your pimples and expect them to go away. You need to apply it to acne-prone areas on your face: cheeks, nose, forehead, chin—wherever your acne is likely to occur. Regular use should keep new pimples from forming—kind of like using crabgrass preventer on your lawn.

Benzoyl peroxide is available OTC at any pharmacy in concentrations from 2.5 to 10 percent. The strength may not matter as much as the formulation: people with dry or sensitive skin will do better with a water-based formulation such as a cream. People with oilier skin usually prefer an alcohol-based preparation such as a gel or lotion, which is more drying.

Benzoyl peroxide is also the active ingredient in the popular Proactiv acne products. As the name suggests, the medication works proactively to prevent pimples rather than to treat them.

Like alcohol, benzoyl peroxide can irritate the skin, especially in higher concentrations. And a few people are allergic, so you might want to try benzoyl peroxide on your arm or wrist first before covering your whole face with it. Beware that benzoyl peroxide will bleach clothing and linens.

The following name-brand products all have benzoyl peroxide as their acne-fighting ingredient:

- Clearasil—various preparations
- Dermalogica Special Clearing Booster
- Neutrogena On-the-Spot Acne Treatment
- Oxy—various preparations
- Persa-Gel 10
- Stridex
- University Medical—acne products
- Zapzyt—various preparations

If one product is irritating or ineffective, try a different brand, or try a salicylic acid preparation, also available OTC and also quite effective against acne. And don't pick your pimples—it didn't help the last one and it won't help the next. If these OTC products are ineffective, see your family doctor to discuss prescription options.

CHAPTER TEN

Save Money Using 10 Over-the-Counter Drugs That Were Once Prescription

91. Harness the heartburn: The H_2s

Once upon a time these drugs were like a miracle.

I still remember when the histamine 2–receptor antagonists came on the market in the 1980s.

I was a medical student—our patient had a bleeding ulcer. He lay there vomiting blood as the acid produced by his own body burned a hole through his stomach. All we could offer him were IVs, painkillers, and a dose of Maalox—and hope he didn't bleed to death.

Then cimetidine (Tagamet) appeared. For the first time, a drug could reduce the amount of acid a person's stomach produces. For ulcer patients, it was life-changing. Finally no more stomach pain, no heartburn, no nausea, vomiting, or hemorrhage.

Cimetidine was followed by ranitidine (Zantac), then nizatidine (Axid) and famotidine (Pepcid)—all prescription drugs, now available in smaller doses over the counter. Initially indicated for true ulcers, these medications are commonly used for milder acid-related stomach problems such as heartburn. And they work great.

These drugs, called H_2-blockers, are not antacids, which neutralize stomach acid on contact. Rather, the H_2-blockers work by entering the bloodstream, eventually reaching the cells of the stomach lining, where they decrease the rate of stomach-acid production.

It is safe to use these drugs for occasional heartburn or acid stomach. It is not a good idea to use them long-term without first consulting your doctor—they may mask a more serious problem, including cancer. Drug interactions are also a concern, especially with cimetidine. The OTC H_2-blockers are inexpensive, but may actually cost less by prescription.

Once Prilosec and "The Purple Pill" hit the market with their advertising campaigns, people tended to forget about the H_2-blockers. Patients don't really understand the difference, anyway, except to say the newer drugs (like Prilosec) work better. "When I take a Prilosec, I can eat anything I want," is a common remark. (Perhaps "eating anything we want" should not be our goal.) And once the patents expired on Tagamet, Zantac, Axid, and Pepcid, the manufacturers dropped their intensive advertising campaigns, allowing their drugs to slip from public awareness.

But all these medications work well and now cost very little. For patients with occasional symptoms, save the cost of an office visit and buy a generic H_2-blocker over the counter for under $10. For patients with ongoing symptoms, see your doctor and read #37 and #92.

92. Reduce your reflux: The PPIs

Americans like their food. (And their alcohol. And their cigarettes.) Some would rather take a pill than give up any of these.

The PPIs are like H_2s on steroids (see #91). Whereas the H_2-blockers decrease stomach acid by about half, the PPIs (proton-pump inhibitors) reduce it about 90 percent.

Once upon a time, patients suffering from acid-related stomach conditions were willing to avoid acid foods like tomatoes and orange juice, spicy foods, fried foods, fatty foods, onions, soda, caffeine, alcohol, tobacco. Even chocolate! Nowadays it seems Americans feel entitled to indulge without bearing the consequences.

It could be the disease has changed—certainly the effect of the ulcer-causing bacteria *Helicobacter pylori* was not recognized 25 years ago. But back then, supersize fries and 32-ounce soft drinks did not exist.

As the inevitable question of health care rationing arises, perhaps lifestyle changes will come into vogue again. But for now, let's consider the drugs.

Assuming one needs medicine for heartburn or an acid stomach, and assuming one does not have a more serious condition such as stomach cancer, then the cheapest way to treat these problems is using the H_2-blockers, discussed in #91. Use an over-the-counter preparation or ask your doctor for something on the $4 list (see #16).

If the H_2-blockers are ineffective, consider a proton-pump inhibitor (PPI). At the time of this writing, both omeprazole (Prilosec) and lansoprazole (Prevacid) are available OTC in low dose for about $25 a month. They remain available by prescription in higher dose—at significantly higher prices: easily $50 to $100 more. (The liquid and oral-disintegrating tablets are available by prescription only.)

Because the OTC versions are so inexpensive compared to the prescription versions, many insurance companies have begun denying payment for this class of medication. Some pharmacies now dispense OTC medication when the doctor writes a prescription for Prilosec or Prevacid.

A word about the best time to take the medicine—those who have heartburn primarily at night may experience more relief taking the medication in the evening. Likewise those with daytime symptoms should take their medicine in the morning. These drugs can be used on an as-needed basis, and probably should be.

Again, if you require daily medication, see your doctor to make sure you don't have a serious condition. If you mask the symptoms of stomach cancer, you won't have saved a dime.

93. Negate your nausea: Meclizine

For the treatment of typical nausea, it's hard to beat meclizine. Curiously, the same strength drug is available either by prescription or over the counter.

Meclizine 25 milligrams is available OTC as:

- Bonine Original
- Dramamine Less Drowsy Formula
- Miscellaneous generics

Meclizine 25 milligrams is available by prescription as:

- Antivert
- Miscellaneous generics

In addition to the 25-milligram dose, the prescription drug (which may actually cost less than the over-the-counter) is available as 12.5 milligrams and 50 milligrams as well.

This medicine should be used short-term to relieve symptoms of an illness that is expected to resolve on its own within a few days, like the stomach flu. It should not be used without consulting your doctor for severe conditions or those that persist.

Nausea is a symptom that may or may not demand medication. Most of us experience nausea—also known as queasiness, or a sick stomach—as part of the stomach flu (viral gastroenteritis). Nausea is often, though not always, a precursor to vomiting. All of us vomit now and then, but the threshold for vomiting varies according to the individual. Some people will feel queasy just reading this paragraph. Most doctors, on the other hand, can discuss blood and guts over dinner without a second thought. Meclizine decreases the sensation of nausea and raises the threshold for vomiting. However, if you're experiencing the stomach flu, staying home in bed a day or two is a good place to start. No sense taking medicine so you can go to work and make your coworkers sick.

Beyond a day or two of vomiting, however, the risk of dehydration sets in. Using meclizine often helps a person keep fluids down (see #49), lowering the risk for excess fluid loss or electrolyte imbalance. Children experiencing vomiting and/or diarrhea become dehydrated more quickly than adults and should be seen by a physician before signs of dehydration appear: listlessness, dry mouth, weight loss, decreased urination. For a patient handout on dehydration visit: www.aafp.org/afp/991201ap/991201a.html.

For people who simply cannot tolerate the sensation of nausea for whatever reason, the drug is quite effective. In a healthy young or middle-aged individual, meclizine may be used to treat:

- Sea sickness
- Car sickness
- Roller coaster sickness
- Air sickness
- Motion sickness
- Nausea due to stomach flu
- Nausea due to irritating foods
- Nausea due to sinus drainage
- Nausea due to certain medications
- Vertigo-type dizziness

It will not help dizziness from other causes, such as low blood pressure or blood loss.

Meclizine may also help persistent nausea, but the cause of such nausea should be established by your doctor before using it on a prolonged basis. Again, you don't want to mask a serious problem by long-term use.

Common side effects of meclizine are drowsiness and dry mouth. If the 25-milligram OTC tablet makes you too drowsy, try half of a chewable tablet. Meclizine may cause urinary retention or blurred vision, or make narrow-angle glaucoma worse. It should not be used during pregnancy, in young children or the elderly without consulting a physician. Otherwise, it is generally safe.

94. Douse the diarrhea: Loperamide

Put the runs on the run with loperamide.

Another example of a medication available both over the counter and by prescription is loperamide, an effective remedy for short-term diarrhea. It comes OTC in a two-milligram dose for adults and a one-milligram liquid preparation for children. The four-milligram dose is available by prescription only. For $5 to $10 you can treat a case of diarrhea at home using the over-the-counter preparation.

Indicated for adults and children over age six, loperamide (Imodium and others) works by slowing the motility of the intestine, allowing more fluid to be absorbed from the stool, thereby producing firmer stools. The most common side effect is constipation, naturally.

Typically, acute diarrhea is caused by intestinal viruses that should resolve on their own within a few days, even without specific treatment. The use of loperamide (or any other antidiarrheal medication) treats only the symptom of loose or watery stools and has little or nothing to do with clearing the virus from the body.

Chronic diarrhea is another problem altogether. Although some people always have loose stools and are not ill, chronic diarrhea may be due to a serious condition, such as inflammatory bowel disease, celiac disease, or even cancer. Consult your doctor before using loperamide beyond a few days, especially if your stools look black, or if you see blood or mucus in them.

In general, diarrhea caused by *Clostridium difficile* ("*C. diff*") or other bacterial infections should not be treated with loperamide. To a degree, having looser stools helps clear these infections (and their associated toxins) from the body. Slowing this process only prolongs the disease.

Clostridium difficile colitis, also known as antibiotic-related colitis, used to be quite rare, seen only in hospitalized patients. Although it continues to be a problem in hospital patients, it is now seen out in the community as well, most commonly in patients who were recently hospitalized, or in any patient who is taking an antibiotic or has done so recently. That's not to say that all antibiotic-related diarrhea is due to this infection. Certain antibiotics are notorious for causing diarrhea, including amoxicillin/clavulanate (Augmentin) and the erythromycin antibiotics. But if the diarrhea persists after discontinuation of the drug, *C. diff*. is a real possibility. Many patients and nurses claim the odor of *C. diff*. diarrhea is especially offensive.

The diagnosis of *Clostridium difficile* colitis is made by obtaining a stool sample for analysis. If you meet the above criteria, call your doctor and plan to bring a specimen with you. (Use a disposable bowl for collection, or place plastic wrap across the toilet bowl so it makes a collection site for the stool. A spoonful or two of feces in a clean jar or disposable plastic container is sufficient. Wear gloves if possible and double-wrap the specimen jar in plastic bags.) The treatment of *Clostridium difficile* colitis is *not* loperamide, but rather a specific antibiotic aimed at the causative organism.

Ask your doctor about whether it's a good idea to use loperamide for traveler's diarrhea. In mild cases it is safe and effective, as is bismuth subsalicylate (Pepto-Bismol). For travel outside the United States, ask your physician if you should bring an antibiotic along (perhaps one from the $4 list). Or check the CDC Web site (www.cdc.gov).

Having loperamide available over the counter allows you to take control of a runaway situation. Remember to see your doctor if the diarrhea lasts more than a few days or if your illness worsens.

95. Say farewell to the flab: Orlistat

With orlistat you can watch the fat go down the drain. Literally.

Unlike other so-called fat-blockers, this one actually works. Try it with a high-fat diet and you'll behold the evidence. The fat goes in one end and comes out the other. You'll see it floating in the commode.

But beware. Sometimes there's leakage.

Normally the intestine absorbs essentially all of the fat in the diet. Orlistat works by inhibiting this process, preventing about a third of dietary fat from being absorbed.

Great! Free calories, you might think. Almost true, but there's a catch.

The body doesn't understand passing fat or oil through the intestine. It treats it like gas, allowing the extra to leak out without alerting the rectal sphincter. All day long we pass a little gas, usually unaware of the occurrence. The same can happen when orlistat blocks the absorption of fat from your diet. The fat leaks out, but it's not invisible. Quite a few of my patients have been dismayed to find an orange-yellow stain on their underwear, or worse yet, on their clothing. It can be quite embarrassing.

For this reason orlistat is intended to be used with a reduced-fat diet, which should not only help the leakage but also reduce your caloric intake. Remember, though, if you block the fat but replace the calories with carbs, you won't lose weight.

Aside from the loose stools and possible leakage, the product poses the potential for loss of fat-soluble vitamins. For this reason patients are advised to take a daily vitamin to make up for any losses. It may also interfere with the absorption of certain medications. If you are on other medications, ask your doctor or pharmacist before beginning orlistat. It is quite unlikely that the amount of fat lost through use of orlistat will make your diet deficient in essential fats.

Usually the weight loss with orlistat is modest, often slower than desired. If we use an 1,800-calorie diet with a third of the calories from fat (600 calories) as an example, 200 calories of fat will be malabsorbed daily. At that rate it would take 18 days to lose one pound. Is it worth $2 to $4 a day to lose maybe two pounds a month? I'll leave that for you to decide.

Orlistat is available by prescription as Xenical (120 mg)

and half-strength over the counter as Alli (60 mg) The OTC costs half as much and works almost as well, with somewhat fewer side effects.

Beware, though, as of 2010 counterfeit Alli has hit the market. To date it has been detected only in product purchased online from questionable sources. It has not been detected in product purchased in drugstores and other retail outlets. For details on detecting the fake product, visit www .myalli.com. The site also links to legitimate online retailers. The counterfeit product does not contain orlistat and, at least in some instances, has been found to contain sibutramine in dangerous amounts.

If your insurance covers weight loss medications ask your doctor for a prescription instead. Otherwise, the OTC is more cost-effective.

96. Abate the ache: The NSAIDs and acetaminophen

NSAIDs are <u>n</u>on<u>s</u>teroidal <u>a</u>nti-<u>i</u>nflammatory <u>d</u>rugs.

As the name suggests, these medications are effective against certain types of inflammation. Symptoms of inflammation include pain, swelling, warmth, and redness. Of these, pain is what usually drives a person to seek medical attention. Arthritis is the prototype inflammatory condition. A badly inflamed joint is red, hot, and swollen, and boy, does it hurt. Think gout.

These drugs are not as powerful as steroids (hence the name), nor do they have as many side effects. Originally all these drugs (except aspirin) were available by prescription only. Now lower strengths are available OTC at very reasonable prices—for example, $10 for 500 generic ibuprofen.

The biggest cost savings in using over-the-counter NSAIDs is the opportunity to treat yourself, thus avoiding the expense of an office call in order to obtain a prescription. Avoiding even one office visit a year would amount to $50 to $100 annually for the self-pay patient.

Conditions that often respond well to over-the-counter NSAIDs, perhaps saving you a trip to the doctor:

- Arthritis, including gout
- Sprained ankles and other sprains
- Back strain and other pulled muscles
- Headaches
- Minor earache
- Stiff neck
- Tendonitis, bursitis, tennis elbow
- Menstrual cramps

The NSAIDs are not advisable for pain associated with stomach or urinary problems, as they sometimes make the problem worse and usually are ineffective for these conditions.

Aspirin works as well as any NSAID, but lasts only a few hours (and probably causes more side effects). Naproxen sodium lasts the longest, often effective 12 to 24 hours. Milligram for milligram, it is the strongest of the three. Ibuprofen lies between the two. Follow package directions for dosing.

The most common side effects are stomach upset, heartburn, and indigestion. The NSAIDs can cause ulcers, even bleeding, in susceptible patients, so ask your doctor before taking them long-term. NSAIDs sometimes cause swelling, or a worsening of high blood pressure, and even drowsiness, especially in the elderly. If you're taking other medications, ask your doctor before using these.

Acetaminophen is not an NSAID but is useful for all these conditions as well, and can be used in combination with the NSAIDs if needed (as in Excedrin). If you're generally a healthy person, the NSAIDs or acetaminophen are worth trying for mild to moderate pain and they won't cost you an arm and a leg.

97. Stifle the sniffles, sneezes, and sleeplessness: The antihistamines

The OTC meds now available to treat your sniffles are basically as good as those by prescription.

In fact, they were available by prescription only, just a few years ago. Now it's possible to treat your allergy and cold symptoms inexpensively and effectively at home without seeing a doctor first. Knowing what's available over the counter and understanding how to use these medications effectively can easily save you hundreds of dollars in just a few years.

This turn of events hasn't made everyone happy. Those of you fortunate enough to have excellent prescription coverage with no co-pay may actually have to pay *more* (than nothing). But with rising prescription co-pays, most insured patients will find the generic OTC formulations very affordable, and uninsured and insured patients alike will be happy to save the cost of an office visit.

Antihistamines dry up secretions, like a runny nose. They don't open up air passages—you'll need a decongestant for that. The combination drugs that have a *D* after their names contain both an antihistamine and a decongestant, like Claritin-D. And with less drainage comes less coughing.

Antihistamines are very useful for itchy conditions as well, such as hives and poison ivy.

The sedating antihistamines are the active ingredient in over-the-counter sleep preparations (Unisom, Tylenol PM, and others). Nonhabit-forming yet effective, the same medicine that keeps you from coughing all night should help you with occasional insomnia.

The OTC *nonsedating antihistamines* are:

- Cetirizine (Zyrtec)
- Loratidine (Claritin)

The OTC *sedating antihistamines* (good for at night) include:

- Chlorpheniramine (many)
- Diphenhydramine (Benadryl)
- Doxylamine (NyQuil)

And what about nose sprays? An alternative to the prescription steroid nasal sprays is cromolyn sodium (NasalCrom), also formerly by prescription only. Not a steroid, it helps prevent the development of allergy symptoms, but is not effective for the same symptoms caused by colds. It is extremely safe, does not cause drowsiness, is not habit-forming, and may be used in combination with any of the oral preparations.

Antihistamine eye drops are also available over the counter for itchy, allergic eyes. Opcon-A and Visine-A both contain the antihistamine pheniramine. Zaditor, once by prescription but now OTC for about $15, contains ketotifen, an antihistamine formerly by prescription only. Check www.zaditor.com for special offers and a link to retailers.

98. Diminish the dandruff: Ketoconazole

For 10 to 20 bucks you can buy a strong antidandruff shampoo that's been medically tested and proven to work, without a prescription.

One-percent ketoconazole antifungal shampoo is now available over the counter. Two-percent ketoconazole shampoo remains available by prescription

So what's the difference? Not much. The prescription product, Nizoral Shampoo (2 percent), simply has twice the active ingredient as the over-the-counter Nizoral A-D Shampoo (1 percent). In some countries outside the United States, the 2 percent product is also available OTC.

Ketoconazole is generally safe to use, though pregnant and nursing women should seek their doctor's advice before using this product due to concerns regarding absorption. Originally ketoconazole came in pill form only, indicated for serious fungal and yeast infections. When the shampoo was developed, it was initially by prescription as well, then later put over the counter.

Ketoconazole is effective against *Pityrosporum ovale*, the organism believed to cause dandruff. By killing the fungus, it eliminates the source of the irritation, thereby allowing your scalp to heal itself.

The shampoo is pleasant, more reminiscent of baby shampoo than medication, and need be used only two or three times a week for good results. The medication kills the fungus, but not instantaneously. Make sure you follow the directions and leave the shampoo on your scalp five minutes before rinsing.

Another scalp condition, common in newborns, is cradle cap. This thick, waxy buildup of dead skin debris occurs primarily on the scalp in the first several months of life. Brushing the scales free with a baby brush and baby shampoo is often effective. Only rarely would a trip to the doctor be necessary for this condition. If you're a first-time parent, ask an experienced relative or neighbor first. Treating the condition is largely a cosmetic issue, but if it's truly bothersome, the OTC Nizoral Shampoo can be helpful. You may want to ask your pediatrician before using the ketoconazole shampoo, especially if your baby has liver problems. Save your time and money, though—just ask at a well-baby check.

The shampoo is useful against a variety of "skin-deep" inflammatory rashes caused by certain fungi and yeasts. The shampoo is officially indicated for dandruff but may be useful in treating athlete's foot, ringworm, tinea versicolor, and the fungal and yeast infections that occur in skin folds. If you know you have any of these skin conditions, it's worth a try using the shampoo to wash the affected body part. If the rash doesn't improve within a week or two, see your doctor to confirm your diagnosis. Some fungal treatments take longer than two weeks to heal, however, and may resolve more quickly with a cream (see #99). The shampoo can be used in conjunction with any topical antifungal preparation.

The one topical fungal condition that ketoconazole *won't* help at all is nail fungus. If you have thick, yellow nails, ask your doctor his or her opinion regarding prescription antifungal medications. They work reasonably well, and with generics now available, the treatment cost is far more affordable than just a few years ago.

99. Finalize the fungus: The antifungals

If the FDA keeps putting all these wonderful drugs over the counter, pretty soon I'll be out of a job.

The nonprescription antifungal and anti-yeast medications are as strong as those by prescription—because they were by prescription not long ago.

First came Monistat. Then Gyne-Lotrimin. Then Lamisil.

Both Monistat (miconazole) and Gyne-Lotrimin (clotrimazole) were originally targeted at vaginal yeast infections and continue to be effective products (miconazole possibly less so due to developing resistance).

Then Lotrimin (like Gyne-Lotrimin, but different name) became available OTC for skin fungal infections such as ringworm, athlete's foot, and jock itch. More recently terbinafine (Lamisil) was placed over the counter for these same conditions. Used according to package directions, these drugs are every bit as effective as prescription creams, and cost only $10 to $20—even less for generics. Tolnaftate (Tinactin) is an older product, also effective, with generics that may cost under $5.

Save the cost of an office visit by treating yourself at home.

A few tips on usage—since fungal rashes tend to recur, I tell my patients to use the medicine until the rash is gone *plus* another week in order to kill off any lingering "invisible" infection.

Also, for *itchy* fungal rashes, a little hydrocortisone will lessen the itching and redness until your body is able to clear the infection. Use the 0.5 or 1.0 percent OTC hydrocortisone cream and apply it at the same time as the antifungal cream. It may be used externally for the itch associated with vaginal yeast infections, but not internally.

The antifungals come not only in creams, but also sprays, powders, and gels—there may be little difference in efficacy but you may find your prefer one product over another. As for shoe sprays and powders, don't expect them to fix your smelly shoes. Cure your skin and get new shoes. Then keep the new shoes dry and wear socks that allow your feet to breathe.

For dozens of pictures of fungal skin rashes, visit Derm-net at:

www.dermnet.com/Tinea-Ringworm-Candidiasis-and-other-Fungal-Infections.

100. Ban the burning: Phenazopyridine

Does it burn when you pee?

This question is directed at women. Men, go see your doctor if you answered yes—it might be something serious.

Among the causes for burning on urination, simple bladder infection is the most common. Kidney stones, sexually transmitted diseases (STDs), and yeast infections may cause burning as well, but these occur with lesser frequency. In women, other symptoms of bladder infection or irritation include frequent urination, nocturia (having to get up at night to urinate), the urgency to get to the bathroom right away, a strong urine odor, and the inability to control urination.

Generally speaking, urinary infections in men are never considered simple. So again, men, if it burns when you pee, see your doctor.

And women, you should see your doctor, too, or at least call her, but there is an over-the-counter remedy that can ease your discomfort until you can do so.

Every week or two, I see a female patient who has sought after-hours care at an emergency room due to burning on urination. Many times they've said they would have waited until morning to see their family doctor if they'd had the pills on hand that "make the burning stop." Too often women are unaware that this medication is available over the counter as well as by prescription. The primary cost savings of Azo lies in avoiding a costly trip to the ER or an urgent care center. Save money by calling or seeing your primary care doctor instead.

If you've ever had a urinary infection, talk to your doctor about what to do when the next one sets in. For some women the answer *will* be to seek care immediately. I, too, have patients who progress rapidly from a simple bladder infection to a full-fledged kidney infection. For the occasional patient with multiple recurrent infections the answer will be to take an antibiotic that your doctor has prescribed for you to keep on hand. But for most women, the answer will be to see your doctor in the morning. In the meantime, phen*azo*pyridine (Azo Standard) will relieve the annoying (or intolerable) burning, sparing you a midnight ER visit. Don't forget to drink extra fluids to help flush the infection from your bladder.

This medication is indicated only for the urgency, frequency, and burning due to *simple* bladder infections, which presupposes you know what that means. If you have a fever, back pain, or vomiting, or feel generally ill, see a doctor right away.

But for the millions of women who've had several bladder infections and know what they are, Azo will relieve your symptoms quickly (within an hour) so you can tolerate the wait until your doctor is available. The OTC preparation is a lower dose of the same medication your doctor might prescribe.

Phenazopyridine does not kill the bacteria that cause urinary infections. It just numbs the bladder and urethra so you don't hurt so badly. *You will still need an antibiotic.* And it turns your urine red or orange. (Tears, too. Contact lenses as well.) To avoid confusing the discoloration with blood, obtain and refrigerate a urine specimen in a clean glass jar *before* you take phenazopyridine. Your doctor can test this in the morning and send it for a culture if necessary.

The reason to refrigerate the specimen is to slow the growth of bacteria. The laboratory diagnosis of urinary tract infection is made based on the number of bacteria present in the urine—there are often a few. But the number of bacteria doubles about every 20–30 minutes in an unrefrigerated specimen. It takes only a few hours for a normal number of bacteria to exceed the threshold where a urinary tract infection is diagnosed. Since there are other causes of burning on urination, you don't want to confuse the issue with a false-positive urine culture.

Remember, if you use Azo and it makes you feel better, that doesn't mean the infection is gone. *You still need to call or see your doctor for an antibiotic.* Don't use this drug to put off seeking medical attention for more than a day or two. But for adult women, it's OK to wait until morning.

A brief word about children—don't use Azo unless you've cleared this with your physician ahead of time. Little girls are much more likely than boys to have bladder infections. Any boy suffering symptoms of a urinary infection should be seen promptly. If your daughter complains of burning but otherwise is playful and acts well, she can probably wait until morning. But if she's just lying around, has a fever, or looks ill, don't wait. You don't want her to require hospitalization for a kidney infection.

CHAPTER ELEVEN

Save Money Using Common Sense

101. Looking back: Thinking ahead

This book has been a journey—30 years for me, perhaps hours for you. Though much has changed since the day I entered medical school, this has remained constant: many Americans have been and continue to be concerned about the cost of health care.

In the last 100 sections we have dealt with ways to navigate the current health care system, imperfect as it is. No doubt the system will change as health reform issues continue to be debated. As the system changes, tactics to save money will need to be adjusted as well.

Taking responsibility for our own health care is the first way to lower costs for each of us as individuals, as well as the nation at large. Thinking ahead would limit expensive trips to the emergency room, mindless accidents, drug and alcohol abuse, sexually transmitted diseases, and many cases of chronic illness.

The point of this book is *not* to be penny-wise and pound-foolish. Skimping on needed medication and treatment usually costs more in the long run. If your doctor writes you an antibiotic, finish it *all* so your symptoms don't return, requiring additional sick days and another trip to the doctor. *Do* go to the doctor when needed—don't wait until you're half-dead and may require hospitalization. *Do* follow the guidelines for when you'll save more money by seeing a doctor than by staying home.

Be a prepared patient. Throughout this book I've detailed ways to interact with your physician in an efficient, cost-effective manner. Organize your thoughts, hopes, and expectations. Medical care is largely an information exchange, and the higher the quality of information your physician has to assess, the better your care.

Don't think of the doctor as "the boss." Think of your physician as a collaborator in your health care. Though your doctor has more medical education than you, you have an equal say in your health care—more so, in fact. It may take some practice—many patients find it difficult to think of themselves as being in charge. But learning to speak up is the key, not only to cost-savings, but to better health care overall.

Consider your body as a pedestrian transportation unit akin to your automobile. You'll want to perform routine maintenance to keep your machine in tip-top condition. You'll want to fix the ding in the windshield before it cracks clear across.

Find a doctor with a servant's heart. Like ministers of faith, healers are called to the profession. Though doctors must charge patients in order to stay in business, if you believe your physician consistently places a higher priority on payment than on service, find another. Your health care will be most efficient if you can maintain an honest, open relationship with someone you trust has your best interest at heart.

For those of you without insurance, I recommend looking into a high-deductible insurance plan. These plans cost significantly less than traditional plans and may be combined with a health savings account. Find an independent insurance agent who can represent a spectrum of options for you.

A high-deductible insurance plan works more like your car insurance or homeowner's insurance. You *will* have to pay for minor expenses (office visits, vaccines, antibiotics), just as you pay for gasoline, new tires, or an oil change. But even if you went to the doctor every month, it's unlikely you'd pay over $1,500 a year in medical expenses. Just as you have car insurance in case you have an unfortunate accident, so your health insurance is in the event of an expensive emergency, such as appendicitis. Expenses above your deductible are covered by insurance. High-deductible insurance plans feature deductibles of $1,000 or more.

A high-deductible plan can easily cost $150 less a month than a traditional plan, money that you could then deposit in a tax-deductible health savings account. As your savings builds, you can convert to an even less expensive higher-deductible plan. With money sitting in your health savings account for health expenditures, you're less likely to forgo doctor visits, medications, eyeglasses, and dental care.

I trust everyone who's read this far has found some way, hopefully many ways, to save money on health care expenses.

Please send your success stories to info@101waystosave moneyonhealthcare.com. And blessings to you and all the members of your health care team.

Appendix 1

Useful Patient-Oriented Internet Resources

Centers for Disease Control and Prevention at www.cdc.gov

The official site of the U.S. Centers for Disease Control and Prevention, the CDC describes their Web site as "Your On-line Source for Credible Health Information."

It includes resources for patients and professionals alike, including the latest information on new health concerns such as the 2009 H1N1 flu outbreak. It is *the* site to visit for travel information including necessary immunizations, environmental health concerns such as asbestos and mold problems, emergency preparedness including bioterrorism, and links to information on numerous common diseases.

For a Spanish version of the same site visit: www.cdc.gov/spanish.

FamilyDoctor.org at www.familydoctor.org

A great place to start, this site is sponsored by the American Academy of Family Physicians. It includes patient-oriented information on hundreds of topics. For more academic information you may visit the parent site, www

.aafp.org, which allows you to search the medical literature and publications.

Links are provided to help you understand your medical bills, your insurance, and Medicare part D, as well as links to various patient assistance programs.

Partnership for Prescription Assistance at www.pparx.com

The Partnership for Prescription Assistance Web site "helps qualifying patients without prescription drug coverage get the medicines they need for free or nearly free," with access to hundreds of public and private programs, including those of nearly 200 pharmaceutical companies. The service is free, available online or by phone (1-888-477-2669), in either English or Spanish.

WebMD at www.webmd.com

Probably the best-known Internet resource for consumer-oriented medical information, WebMD offers a symptom checker, a physician directory, a hospital locator, and up-to-date information on numerous health conditions and tests. It also allows you to establish an online personal health record.

The Merck Manual Medical Library at www.merck.com/mmhe/index.html

Respected for generations, the Merck Manual has long been a standard reference for physicians around the world. Now an online version exists, written in everyday language, to help laymen and professionals understand medical symptoms, disorders, diagnosis, treatment, prognosis, and prevention. Merck & Co., Inc. provide the online manual as a public service.

The Mayo Clinic at www.mayoclinic.com

"Medical information and tools for healthy living." This site includes an abundance of information on a wide variety of topics, including beautiful multimedia presentations. They also offer the Mayo Clinic Health Manager to store your health data in a free online Microsoft HealthVault account, which you can share with others you trust, such as family members and health professionals.

National Institutes of Health at www.nih.com

According to their mission statement, "NIH is the steward of medical and behavioral research for the Nation." Look here for information regarding research on diseases of concern to you or your family, especially unusual conditions.

MedScape at www.medscape.com

Primarily a learning center, this Web site allows the public limited access to search medical journals and articles. Physicians and other health care professionals may register for a free account with access to continuing medical education and journal articles.

Appendix 2

Pharmaceutical Sites with Offers for OTC Medications

Web site	Product	Purpose
www.advil.com	Advil, Advil PM	Pain, fever
www.afrin.com	Afrin	Nasal congestion
www.alavert.com	Alavert, Alavert-D	Allergies
www.aleve.com	Aleve products	Pain, fever
www.anbesol.com	Anbesol	Cold sores
www.azoproducts.com/buy/coupon	Azo products	Urinary pain
www.benadryl.com/#/Coupons	Benadryl	Allergies
www.caltrate.com	Caltrate	Calcium replacement
www.chlortrimeton.com	Chlor-trimeton	Allergies
www.claritin.com	Claritin, Claritin-D	Allergies

Web site	Product	Purpose
www.clearasil.us	Clearasil products	Acne
www.dimetapp.com	Dimetapp products	Colds, allergies
www.drscholls.com/ drscholls/wartremoval.jsp	Dr. Scholl's Freeze Away	Wart remover
www.imodium.com	Imodium products	Diarrhea
www.lotrimin.com	Lotrimin products	Antifungal, anti-yeast
www.miralax.com/miralax/ consumer/savenow.jsp	MiraLax	Constipation
www.monistat.com/ monistat-1-day	Monistat products	Anti-yeast cream
www.myalli.com	Alli (orlistat)	Weight loss
www.nasalcrom.com/ offers.php	Nasalcrom nose spray	Nasal allergies
www.pepcid.com	Pepcid, Pepcid Complete	Acid reflux, heartburn
www.prevacid24hr.com	Prevacid24HR	Acid reflux, heartburn
www.prilosecotc.com/en_ US/consumer	Prilosec	Acid reflux, heartburn
www.ridlice.com	Rid products	Head lice
www.tagamet.com	Tagamet	Acid reflux, heartburn

Web site	Product	Purpose
www.tinactin.com	Tinactin products	Antifungal
www.tylenol.com	Tylenol products	Pain, fever
www.zaditor.com	Zaditor	Eye allergy
www.zapzyt.com/home	Zapzyt	Acne
www.zegerid.com	Zegerid	Acid reflux, heartburn
www.zyrtec.com	Zyrtec, Zyrtec-D	Colds, allergies

Appendix 3

Pharmaceutical Sites with Offers for Prescription Drugs

Web site	Product	Purpose
www.abreva.com	Abreva	Cold sores
www.aciphex.com	AcipHex	Heartburn/GERD
www.actonel.com	Actonel	Osteoporosis
www.actos.com/actos/specialoffers.aspx	Actos, Actoplusmet, Duetact	Diabetes Type II
www.advair.com	Advair Diskus	Asthma and COPD
www.aggrenox.com	Aggrenox	Stroke prevention
www.allegra.com	Allegra, Allegra-D	Allergies
www.alphaganp.com/Patient/Default.aspx	Alphagan P	Glaucoma
www.altabax.com	Altabax	Skin infection/impetigo

Web site	Product	Purpose
www.amitiza.com	Amitiza	Constipation, irritable bowel
www.amrix.com/pat/default.aspx	Amrix	Muscle relaxer
www.apidra.com/default.aspx	Apidra	Diabetes
www.aplenzin.com/default.aspx	Aplenzin	Depression
www.asmanex.com/asmanex/application	Asmanex	Asthma controller drug
www.avandia.com	Avandia or Avandamet	Diabetes Type II
www.avodart.com	Avodart	Enlarged prostate
www.axert.com/axert	Axert	Migraine headache
www.boniva.com	Boniva	Osteoporosis
www.caduet.com	Caduet	Hypertension + high cholesterol
www.chantix.com/index.aspx	Chantix	Smoking cessation
www.cialis.com	Cialis	Erectile dysfunction
www.clarinex.com	Clarinex	Allergies

Web site	Product	Purpose
www.colcrys.com/patient-assistance-program.htm	Colcrys	Gout
www.coregcr.com	Coreg CR	Heart, hypertension
www.crestor.com/c/home.aspx	Crestor	High cholesterol
www.cymbalta.com	Cymbalta	Depression
www.dexilant.com	Dexilant	Acid reflux
www.differin.com	Differin	Acne
www.diovan.com/index.jsp	Diovan	Hypertension
www.enablex.com	Enablex	Overactive bladder
www.enbrel.com	Enbrel	Inflammatory arthritis
www.femara.com	Femara	Breast cancer prevention
www.flector.com	Flector patch	Arthritis patch
www.foradil.com	Foradil	Asthma and COPD
www.4flomax.com/mof/basics.jsp	Flomax	Enlarged prostate
www.frova.com	Frova	Migraine headache

Web site	Product	Purpose
www.januvia.com	Januvia	Diabetes
www.keppraxr.com	Keppra XR	Epilepsy
www.levitra.com	Levitra	Erectile dysfunction
www.lialda.com	Lialda	Ulcerative colitis
www.lidoderm.com	Lidoderm	Pain after shingles
www.lipitor.com	Lipitor	High cholesterol
www.lovenox.com/consumer/default.aspx	Lovenox	Blood clots
www.lumigan.com	Lumigan	Glaucoma
www.lunesta.com	Lunesta	Insomnia
www.maxairautohalercoupon.com	Maxair	Asthma
www.maxalt.com	Maxalt	Migraine headache
www.us.micardis.com	Micardis	High blood pressure
www.mirapex.com/pd	Mirapex	Parkinson's disease

Web site	Product	Purpose
www.mysymbicort.com	Symbicort	Asthma and COPD
www.nascobal.com	Nascobal	Vitamin B_{12} deficiency
www.nasonex.com/nasx/application	Nasonex	Nasal allergies
www.nuvaring.com	NuvaRing	Contraception
www.omnaris.com	Omnaris	Nasal allergies
www.onglyza.com	Onglyza	Diabetes Type II
www.oxistat.com	Oxistat	Acne
www.pataday.com	Pataday	Eye allergies
www.pristiq.com	Pristiq	Depression
www.propecia.com	Propecia	Male pattern hair loss
www.proventilhfa.com	Proventil	Asthma and COPD
www.purplepill.com	Nexium	Heartburn/GERD
www.relpax.com	Relpax	Migraine headache
www.restasis.com	Restasis	Chronic dry eyes

Web site	Product	Purpose
www.singulair.com	Singulair	Asthma and allergies
www.skelaxin.com	Skelaxin	Muscle spasm
www.toviaz.com	Toviaz	Overactive bladder
www.trilipix.com	Trilipix	High triglycerides
www.twinject.com	Twinject	Emergency allergy treatment (bee sting allergy)
www.uroxatral.com	Uroxatral	Enlarged prostate
www.vaniqa.com	Vaniqa	Unwanted facial hair in women
www.ventolin.com	Ventolin	Asthma and COPD
www.veramyst.com	Veramyst	Nasal allergies
www.vesicare.com	VESIcare	Overactive bladder
www.voltarengel.com	Voltaren gel	Arthritis
www.vytorin.com	Vytorin	High cholesterol

Web site	Product	Purpose
www.vyvanseadult.com	Vyvanse	Adult ADHD
www.xyzal.com	Xyzal	Allergies
www.yaz-us.com	Yaz	Contraception
www.zanaflex.com/consumer/Default.aspx	Zanaflex	Spasticity
www.zegerid.com	Zegerid	Acid reflux
www.zetia.com	Zetia	High cholesterol

Addenda:

This list is merely a sampling of available offers, all of which are subject to change without notice. Restrictions may apply. Each offer requires a valid prescription.

For drugs not listed, try looking for www.*[enter-drug-name-here]*.com.

In addition to these coupon offers and rebates, many manufacturer Web sites offer assistance programs for uninsured or underinsured patients.

Most of these offers can be used toward prescription co-pays for insured patients, as well as toward the full cost of the medication for uninsured individuals.

Appendix 4

Pharmacies with Generics
for About $4 a Month

Store Name and Region	Web site
Acme (OH)	www.acmestores.com/400-prescriptions.php
CVS (Nationwide) ($9.99 for 90 days with Savings Pass)	www.cvs.com
Discount Drug Mart (OH)	www.discount-drugmart.com/rxlistall.asp
Family Fare Supermarkets (MI)	www.familyfaresupermarkets.com
Food City (KY, VA, TN)	www.foodcity.com/pharmacy
Fred Meyer (AK, ID, OR, WA)	www.fredmeyer.com/generic/Pages/alpha_listing.aspx
Giant Eagle (OH, PA, WV)	www.gianteagle.com/pharmacy/home
Good Neighbor Pharmacy (Nationwide)	www.gnppsc.com/downloads/GNPPN_Generic_30-day.pdf

Store Name and Region	Web site
Hy-Vee (Midwest)	www.hy-vee.com/health/ pharmacy/generics/default .aspx
Kinney Drugs (NY, VT)	www.kinneydrugs.com/ pharmacy/discount -prescription-plan.html
Kmart (Nationwide) ($5)	www.kmart.com/shc/s/ dap_10151_10104_DAP_ Kmart+Pharmacy+Generics+5
Kroger (Nationwide)	www.kroger.com/generic/ Pages/default.aspx
Marc's (NE Ohio)	www.marcs.com/copy_rx399 .cfm
Sam's Club (Nationwide) (store membership required)	www.samsclub.com/ pharmacy
Target (Nationwide)	www.sites.target.com/site/en/ health/generic_drugs .jsp?sort=alph
Walgreens (Nationwide) $12 for 90 days (membership required)	www.walgreens.com
Walmart (Nationwide)	www.i.walmartimages.com/i/ if/hmp/fusion/customer_list .pdf
Wegmans (Nationwide)	www.wegmans.com

This list is subject to change without notice.

Appendix 5

Internet Sites for Medical School Financing

Already America needs more primary care doctors, with the physician shortage expected to increase in coming years.

According to the *New York Times*, December 2008, the median cost for one year of medical school is $44,000 for state residents at public schools and $62,000 at private schools, for a whopping total of about $200,000 in medical school expenses. Even with a good income, school loans of this amount take decades to repay.

This huge debt load is driving doctors out of primary care. Though it takes a few more years of training to become a highly paid specialist, the large difference in income is enticing medical students away from family practice, pediatrics, and internal medicine.

Not coming from a wealthy background, I financed three years of my medical education through the National Health Service Corps. In return I worked three years in a designated doctor shortage area in Appalachian Kentucky.

The following references are provided for medical and premedical students, interested in entering primary care, but lacking the financial means.

National Health Service Corps

The NHSC is "committed to improving the health of the nation's underserved communities."

The corps offers scholarships to medical students (dentists, nurse practitioners, nurse midwives, and physician assistants as well) willing to serve as primary care providers in underserved communities (one year of service for each year of scholarship with a minimum of two years). In addition to school expenses, they provide a (taxable) monthly stipend for living expenses ($1,269 a month in 2009–2010). Loan repayment programs are available as well, currently up to $50,000. Having participated in the National Health Service Corps myself, I can attest to the worthiness of this long-established program.

NHSC: http://nhsc.bhpr.hrsa.gov

Military Health Care Scholarships

Similarly structured, these scholarships pay for medical school and offer a monthly stipend for living expenses (approximately $1,992/month in 2010). They require military service upon completion of medical training, generally one year of service for each year of scholarship.

Army: www.goarmy.com/amedd/hpsp.jsp

Navy: www.navy.com/careers/healthcare/physician.html

Air Force: www.airforce.com/opportunities/healthcare/education

Various Opportunities and Scholarships

Cuba

The Latin American School of Medicine in Havana, Cuba
Intended for U.S. students committed to practicing medicine in poor and underserved U.S. communities after graduation. For information visit: www.ifconews.org/node/411.

New York

Doctors Across New York
Loan repayment awards up to $150,000 in exchange for working in primary care in an underserved community in the state of New York. Brochure available at www.health.state .ny.us/professionals/doctors/graduate_medical_education/ doctors_across_ny.

Texas

Texas Higher Education Coordinating Board
Physician Education Loan Repayment Program
Loan repayment awards up to $160,000 in exchange for working in primary care in an underserved Texas community. Information available at www.dshs.state.tx.us/chpr/ PELRP.shtm.

Ohio

Ohio Physician Loan Repayment Program
Up to $80,000 of medical school debt repaid over four years in exchange for practicing in a Health Professional

Shortage Area in Ohio. Details at www.explorehealthcareers
.org/en/Funding.56.aspx.

U.S.A.

Information on loan forgiveness programs in various states
including: Arizona, Virginia, West Virginia, Oklahoma,
North Carolina, Nebraska, New Mexico, New Hampshire,
New Jersey, Rhode Island, Kentucky, Minnesota, Washington
state, and Wisconsin.

Details at www.explorehealthcareers.org/en/FundingSearch
.aspx.

Index